MONOGRAPH
EPILEPSY

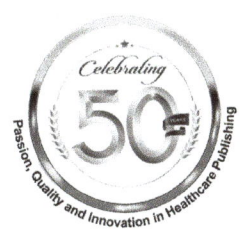

MONOGRAPH
EPILEPSY

Editors

Rajesh Shankar Iyer MD DM (Neuro) FRCP (Glasgow)
Senior Consultant
Neurophysician and Epileptologist
Kovai Medical Center and Hospitals
Coimbatore, Tamil Nadu, India

Mugundhan Krishnan MD DM (Neuro) FRCP (Glasgow)
FRCP (London) FRCP (Ireland) FACP (USA) FICP
Professor and Head
Department of Neurology
Government Stanley Medical College
Chennai, Tamil Nadu, India

Forewords

BA Muruganathan

AV Srinivasan

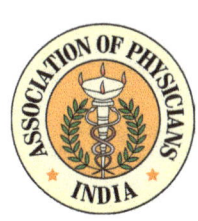
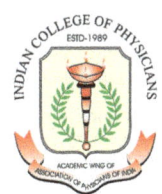

Under the Auspices of Indian College of
Physicians, Academic Wing of
the Association of Physicians of India

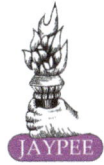

JAYPEE BROTHERS MEDICAL PUBLISHERS
The Health Sciences Publisher
New Delhi | London

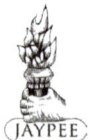 **Jaypee Brothers Medical Publishers (P) Ltd**

Headquarters
Jaypee Brothers Medical Publishers (P) Ltd
4838/24, Ansari Road, Daryaganj
New Delhi 110 002, India
Phone: +91-11-43574357
Fax: +91-11-43574314
Email: jaypee@jaypeebrothers.com

Overseas Offices
J.P. Medical Ltd
83 Victoria Street, London
SW1H 0HW (UK)
Phone: +44 20 3170 8910
Fax: +44 (0)20 3008 6180
Email: info@jpmedpub.com

Website: www.jaypeebrothers.com
Website: www.jaypeedigital.com

© 2020 Indian College of Physicians, Academic Wing of Association of Physicians of India.

The views and opinions expressed in this book are solely those of the original contributor(s)/author(s) and do not necessarily represent those of editor(s) of the book.

All rights reserved. No part of this publication may be reproduced, stored or transmitted in any form or by any means, electronic, mechanical, photocopying, recording or otherwise, without the prior permission in writing of the publishers.

All brand names and product names used in this book are trade names, service marks, trademarks or registered trademarks of their respective owners. The publisher is not associated with any product or vendor mentioned in this book.

Medical knowledge and practice change constantly. This book is designed to provide accurate, authoritative information about the subject matter in question. However, readers are advised to check the most current information available on procedures included and check information from the manufacturer of each product to be administered, to verify the recommended dose, formula, method and duration of administration, adverse effects and contraindications. It is the responsibility of the practitioner to take all appropriate safety precautions. Neither the publisher nor the author(s)/editor(s) assume any liability for any injury and/or damage to persons or property arising from or related to use of material in this book.

This book is sold on the understanding that the publisher is not engaged in providing professional medical services. If such advice or services are required, the services of a competent medical professional should be sought.

Every effort has been made where necessary to contact holders of copyright to obtain permission to reproduce copyright material. If any have been inadvertently overlooked, the publisher will be pleased to make the necessary arrangements at the first opportunity. The **CD/DVD-ROM** (if any) provided in the sealed envelope with this book is complimentary and free of cost. **Not meant for sale.**

Inquiries for bulk sales may be solicited at: jaypee@jaypeebrothers.com

Monograph: Epilepsy / Rajesh Shankar Iyer, Mugundhan Krishnan

First Edition: 2020

ISBN: 978-93-86261-42-7

Contributors

Editors

Rajesh Shankar Iyer MD DM (Neuro) FRCP (Glasgow)
Senior Consultant
Neurophysician and Epileptologist
Kovai Medical Center and Hospitals
Coimbatore, Tamil Nadu, India

Mugundhan Krishnan MD DM (Neuro) FRCP (Glasgow) FRCP (London) FRCP (Ireland) FACP (USA) FICP
Professor and Head
Department of Neurology
Government Stanley Medical College
Chennai, Tamil Nadu, India

Contributing Authors

Neeraj N Baheti DM
Consultant Neurologist and Epileptologist
Department of Neurology
Dr GM Taori Central India Institute of Medical Sciences
Nagpur, Maharashtra, India

Biji Bahuleyan MCh
Consultant
Department of Neurology
Kerala Institute of Medical Sciences
Trivandrum, Kerala, India

Atma Ram Bansal DM
Consultant
Department of Neurology
Medanta-The Medicity
Gurgaon, Haryana, India

Ajith Cherian DM
Assistant Professor
Department of Neurology
Sree Chitra Tirunal Institute for Medical Sciences and Technology
Trivandrum, Kerala, India

Haseeb Hassan DM
Post Doctoral Fellow in Epilepsy
Consultant Neurologist and Epileptologist
Rabindranath Tagore International Institute of Cardiac Sciences
Kolkata, West Bengal, India

Divya KP DM
Department of Neurology
Sree Chitra Tirunal Institute for Medical Sciences and Technology
Trivandrum, Kerala, India

Ramshekhar N Menon MD DNB DM
Consultant
Department of Neurology
R Madhavan Nayar Centre for
Comprehensive Epilepsy Care
Sree Chitra Tirunal Institute for
Medical Sciences and Technology
Trivandrum, Kerala, India

Harsh Patel DCH DNB DM
Consultant
Department of Neurology
Zydus Hospital
Ahmedabad, Gujarat, India

Shiva Kumar R DM
Senior Consultant
Epileptologist and Neurologist
Institute of Neurosciences
Sakra World Hospital
Bengaluru, Karnataka, India

Ashalatha Radhakrishnan DM
Additional Professor
R Madhavan Nayar Centre for
Comprehensive Epilepsy Care
Sree Chitra Tirunal Institute for
Medical Sciences and Technology
Trivandrum, Kerala, India

Suvasini Sharma MD DM
Associate Professor
Department of Pediatrics
Lady Hardinge Medical College
New Delhi, India

Foreword

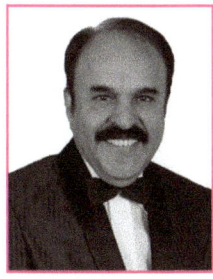

BA Muruganathan
MD FRCP (Glasgow, London, Ireland) FACP (USA) FPCP (Philippines) FICP
Dean, Indian College of Physicians (ICP), 2016–17
Governor Elect, American College of Physicians (ACP) India Chapter
President, Hypertension Society of India (HSI), 2015–16
President, Association of Physicians of India (API), 2013–14
Emeritus Professor, The Tamil Nadu Dr MGR Medical University
Chairman, AG Hospital
Tirupur, Tamil Nadu, India

Epilepsy is one of the most common problems encountered by the practising physician in his day to day practice. There are plenty of problems and pitfalls in the current clinical practice of epilepsy. This results in various errors in the identification, evaluation, and management of this intriguing disease. Epilepsy may be diagnosed in some when they actually do not have the disease and vice versa. The practising clinician is many a time uncertain as to when a diagnostic test is to be done and what is the ideal test for the given candidate. Anti-epileptic drugs may be inappropriately chosen and inadequately administered. Drug resistant epilepsy may not be identified sufficiently early. The benefits of epilepsy surgery are not yet sufficiently recognized and understood by the community level practitioner. Women with epilepsy may not get proper guidance and counseling to handle marriage, pregnancy, and motherhood. The myths surrounding the disease are not making life easier for the unfortunate patient with epilepsy.

The past two decades have seen plenty of developments in the diagnosis and management of epilepsy. Video electroencephalogram is now widely used and helps to separate the mimickers from epilepsy. Various refinements in magnetic resonance imaging techniques have come to precisely identify the seizure focus. The sophisticated investigatory modalities like positron emission tomography and single-photon emission computed tomography are more freely available than before. More centers have come up in India with dedicated care for epilepsy and more epilepsy surgeries are currently being performed.

This monograph edited by Dr Rajesh Shankar Iyer and Dr Mugundhan Krishnan comprehensively covers the clinically relevant and common problem of epilepsy. All the 10 chapters have been carefully chosen addressing the various pitfalls mentioned above. The authors have done a wonderful job by succinctly elucidating the topics making it highly appealing to the practitioner.

I am sure this initiative by the editors will bridge the information gap of the treating physician, with regard to epilepsy and help them practice epilepsy in a more evidence based manner. I congratulate Dr Iyer and Dr Krishnan for successfully bringing out this monograph which is a must read for all practising physicians.

Foreword

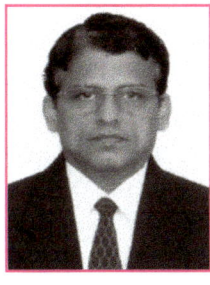

AV Srinivasan
MD DM PhD (Neuro) DSc FRCP (London) FAAN FIAN
Emeritus Professor
The Tamil Nadu Dr MGR Medical University
President
Indian Academy of Neurology

I am extremely pleased and honored to write this foreword for this easy paced monograph on epilepsy.

I extend my heartfelt congratulations to Dr Rajesh Shankar Iyer, Dr Mugundhan Krishnan, and their colleagues for putting together this brilliant monograph on epilepsy. The topic selection and presentations have been very appropriate and is written in simple prose and presented succinctly touching all the relevant aspects of epilepsy. This provides an excellent introduction to epilepsy of the past, present, and future. The chapters on classification of epilepsy, epilepsy mimics, and diagnosis of epilepsy give an excellent observation sense. An approach to adult with the first unprovoked seizure and women with epilepsy explicitly express the word sense. The sheer brilliance of common sense is exquisitely seen in drug resistant epilepsy and status epilepticus in adults. The clinical sense provided in epilepsy surgery is clear and concise.

I have no doubt that this monograph on epilepsy should be in the bookshelves of every neurophysician, neurosurgeon, physician, and in medical libraries of all institutions of neurosciences.

Preface

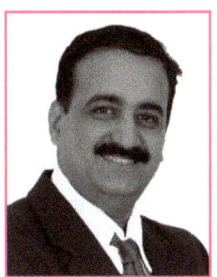

Rajesh Shankar Iyer
MD DM (Neuro) FRCP (Glasgow)

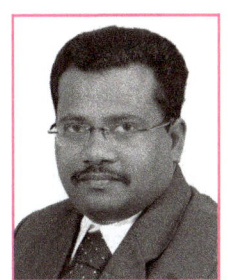

Mugundhan Krishnan
MD DM (Neuro) FRCP (Glasgow) FRCP (London)
FRCP (Ireland) FACP (USA) FICP

Epilepsy is a chronic disorder with lot of peculiarities. It is not a joke to live with the fear of getting an attack of seizure any time. One might also get perturbed by the thought of the adverse effects of anti-epileptic drugs taken indefinitely. It is one of those disorders where the quality of life may get severely compromised. It could interfere with driving; adversely affect employment and marriage possibilities. Psychiatric comorbidities are common including disorders of mood and affect. Social stigma and ill-conceived beliefs about the disease make the treatment extremely difficult.

Learning of any disease is incomplete without proper understanding of the history and epilepsy is no exception. The introductory chapter "Epilepsy: Past, Present, and Future" touches upon the past, discusses the present state, and outlines the future prospects for the disease. When dealing with recurrent seizures, one should move from seizure to syndrome, i.e., try and make a syndromic diagnosis. This would enable to choose the appropriate treatment and more importantly prognosticate better. Hence, the various seizures and the syndromes are lucidly brought out in the second chapter, "Epilepsy Classification: Seizures and Syndromes".

One of the major pitfalls while managing the disease is failure to recognize the nonepileptic conditions. These mimickers are well described in the third chapter "Epilepsy Mimics". One should take all efforts to avoid this mistake considering the huge psychosocial burden associated with the diagnosis of epilepsy. Proper history and video electroencephalogram recording would help us in this regard. With the advent of technology, the treating physician is now bombarded with an array of investigatory modalities. Which one to choose in which situation is well discussed in the fourth chapter, "Epilepsy Diagnosis". That these advanced technological initiatives are bound to fail without a proper history taking is emphasized by the author in no uncertain terms.

Dealing with the first episode of seizure is different from that of dealing with recurrent seizures. We are unsure whether it is a one-off incident or there are many more seizures to follow. The guidelines to follow while evaluating and treating the first seizure episode have been discussed in the fifth chapter, "Approach to the First Episode of Seizure". In the good old days of practice, only phenytoin, phenobarbitone, carbamazepine, and sodium valproate were available for the treatment of epilepsy. Nowadays the market is flooded with newer anti-epileptic drugs, thereby giving the physician plenty of options. On the flip side, more caution need to be exercised in drug selection as one should ensure suitability of the drug for the syndrome. Dose titration should be carefully done as some drugs show adverse effects only with faster titration. One should be aware of the ideal anti-epileptic drug for comorbid medical conditions and the drug interactions. These issues have been well addressed in the sixth chapter, "Epilepsy Pharmacotherapy: The Anti-epileptic Drugs".

Women suffering from epilepsy have unique issues with regard to marriage, contraception, fertility, and childbearing. You can read the seventh chapter "Epilepsy and Women" to get a good overview as to how to help them through these situations. One of the major challenges while handling epilepsy is the partial or total unresponsiveness to drugs. When seizures do not respond to drugs, the quality of life of the individual and, therefore, of the entire family gets jeopardized. An evidence based approach to drug resistant epilepsy highlighting the latest trends in its management is available in the eighth chapter, "Drug Resistant Epilepsy".

Status epilepticus is the other major challenge faced by emergency physicians. The outcome in a status depends on the etiology and also on how fast one is able to arrest the seizures and hence it is a medical emergency. Of late, the new entity called super-refractory status has come in vogue wherein the status continues beyond 24 hours and new treatment modalities are being recommended for control of seizures in this situation. The etiology in super refractory status is mostly unknown though autoimmune epilepsy syndromes are being increasingly blamed. I am sure the ninth chapter "Status Epilepticus: The Current Status" would make a very interesting and informative reading.

Epilepsy surgery comes as a boon for those unfortunate patients who fail to respond to drugs but are fortunate to have a surgically remediable syndrome. Only a few with drug resistant epilepsy become eligible for surgery and hence are deemed surgically privileged. Unfortunately, this treatment modality has failed to permeate and reach the masses. Misconceptions persist not only among general practitioners and physicians but even among the specialist population. For all these reasons, epilepsy surgery remains the most underutilized among all the available therapeutic strategies today leaving a big surgical treatment gap in the community. This gap is the difference between the surgically eligible candidates and those who really undergo surgery. This situation is akin to what prevailed in the society three decades ago when cardiac surgery opening the chest wall was introduced as a coronary revascularization technique. It is time the society at large, and the clinician in particular, recognize epilepsy surgery for the appropriately selected candidate as a life changing treatment modality improving the quality of life by leaps and bounds. All the various surgical treatments currently available are discussed in the last chapter, "Epilepsy Surgery".

It is thus clear that epilepsy means more than recurrent seizures. When dealing with such a chronic disorder of wider ramifications, the physician should be well equipped in handling the vagaries. We have conceived the chapters and brought out this monograph with the sole idea of facilitating the medical practitioner dealing with epilepsy on a daily basis. We profusely thank all the contributing authors who despite their busy schedule came forward and contributed immensely towards this theme. We hope our efforts will enable the physician to approach, investigate and treat epilepsy more confidently and in an evidence based manner.

Happy and enjoyable reading to one and all.

Rajesh Shankar Iyer
Mugundhan Krishnan

Contents

1. **Epilepsy: Past, Present, and Future** 1
   Haseeb Hassan

2. **Epilepsy Classification: Seizures and Syndromes** 9
   Ajith Cherian, Divya KP

3. **Epilepsy Mimics** 18
   Suvasini Sharma, Harsh Patel

4. **Epilepsy Diagnosis** 26
   Shiva Kumar R

5. **Approach to the First Episode of Seizure** 47
   Rajesh Shankar Iyer

6. **Epilepsy Pharmacotherapy: The Anti-epileptic Drugs** 51
   Mugundhan Krishnan

7. **Epilepsy and Women** 67
   Neeraj N Baheti, Atma Ram Bansal

8. **Drug-resistant Epilepsy** 76
   Rajesh Shankar Iyer

9. **Status Epilepticus: The Current Status** 86
   Ramshekhar N Menon, Ashalatha Radhakrishnan

10. **Epilepsy Surgery** 104
    Biji Bahuleyan

CHAPTER 1

Epilepsy: Past, Present, and Future

Haseeb Hassan

INTRODUCTION

The epilepsy is as old as mankind. The universal misbelief of the condition caused by "divine curse" and remedy directed to please the "supernatural forces" dominated till 18th century. The scientific understanding of epilepsy in last two centuries has given way to many path-breaking discoveries, developments and interventions. This chapter reviews the historical progress in field of epileptology, the present understanding, the current unmet needs in epilepsies and future developments that is likely to improve the understanding and management of epilepsies.

UNDERSTANDING EPILEPSY: PAST, PRESENT, AND FUTURE

The existence of epilepsy is known to human civilization from as early as 2000 BC. Descriptions of epileptic fits are available in all ancient civilization and evils, ghost and supernatural factors were believed to be the reason in almost all ancient civilization.[1] In Ayurvedic texts, epilepsy has been mentioned as *Apasmara* or *Apasmrti*. There is a detailed description of epilepsy in the *Charaka Samhita*. It was attributed to *dosa* (humor) and treatment ranging from *mantra* (hymn), emesis, purgative, topical application and oral medications were used.[2]

Till 19th century, there was no serious challenge to supernatural theory, though time to time, possibility of epilepsy being disorder of body and mind was put forward by many famous ancient physicians, Hippocrates being most prominent. French and British medical schools by end of 18th century and beginning of 19th century started to understand epilepsy as brain disorder. Both observational study and animal experiments were carried out and anti-epileptic property of Bromide was discovered. John Hughling Jackson (1835–1911), Father of epileptology laid the foundation of scientific basis of epilepsy.[3] Jackson studied epilepsy on a pathological and anatomical basis and postulated origin of epilepsy from damaged cortex in case of focal epilepsy. Gowers published his famous book The Borderlands of Epilepsy[4] recognizing the mimickers of epilepsy. During the 1920s, Lennox (1884–1960) and Cobb (1887–1968) focused on the effects of starvation, ketogenic diet and altered cerebral oxygen in seizures and published their first monograph entitled "Epilepsy from the Standpoint of Physiology and Treatment".[1] In 1941, Jasper (1906–1999) and Kershman proved that the temporal lobe is the site of origin of psychomotor seizures.[5] Graham Goddard demonstrated changes in hippocampus causes by electrical stimulus and mechanism of "epileptogenesis", the process in which the normal brain is transformed into one that generates seemingly unprovoked seizure and coined the term "kindling".[6]

In last few decades, tremendous progress has been made in understanding pathophysiology of epilepsy, mechanism of epileptogenesis, various etiologies and genetics of epilepsy. Role of neurotransmitters and imbalance between excitatory and inhibitory neurotransmitters is researched in last 50 years. International League Against Epilepsy (ILAE) in 1969 proposed first classification of epileptic disorders based on seizure type, electroencephalography (EEG) characteristics, anatomical substrate, etiology and the age.[7] The concept of electroclinical syndrome emerged subsequently. Further exponential development in genetics led to discovery of several monogenic epilepsies and numerous susceptibility genes. These developments were incorporated by ILAE to propose new classification in 2010.[8]

The focus has now extended beyond "seizures". Psychiatric and cognitive comorbidities that were earlier considered as consequence of epilepsy or anti-epileptic drugs (AEDs) is being recognized as part of disorder that can pre-exist or coexist and are probably caused by common denominator with additional influence of psychosocial factors and medications. The neurobiological mechanism of these psychiatric manifestations is still very poorly understood and its correlation with seizure seems to be poor though some correlation with interictal epileptiform discharges has been observed especially in Benign rolandic epilepsy[9] and its spectrum extending to Landau-Kleffner syndrome. The understanding of complex interplay between psychiatric comorbidities and cognitive disability with epilepsy, EEG abnormalities and its underlying mechanisms is at very nascent stage and needs future research.

Understanding underlying mechanism of epileptogenesis and its evolution from cellular, molecular to level of circuits and network is another key area of future research. The term "epileptogenesis" refers to the process by which normal brain tissue is transformed into tissue capable of generating spontaneous seizures. This area is looked forward as potential target to cure epilpesy.[10]

ELECTROENCEPHALOGRAPHY AND OTHER DIAGNOSTIC TOOL FOR EPILEPSY: EVOLUTION AND FUTURE TREND

There are many references of animal experiments on effect of electrical stimulation of brain and spontaneous electrical activity of brain.[1] In 1929, Berger (1873–1941), a German neurologist, reported his findings on human brainwaves. In 1932 and 1933, he described postictal changes and 3-Hz spike and wave discharges. He made important observations on patients and on healthy subjects over the next few years. His work on EEG was carried forward by Frederic Andrews Gibbs (1903–1992), an American neurologist, and Erna Leonhardt Gibbs (1904–1987), technician and wife of Frederic, who in collaboration with Lennox, established the correlation between EEG findings and epileptic convulsions.[11] Gibbs couple published in 1941 their monumental monograph "Atlas of Electroencephalography".[12] Henri Jean Pascal Gastaut (1915–1995) discovered photic stimulation as activation procedure. He also described lambda waves, pi rhythm, mu rhythm, rolandic spikes and posterior theta rhythm. He described two epilepsy syndromes under his name, Gastaut-type idiopathic childhood occipital epilepsy and Lennox-Gastaut syndrome.[1]

The technology of EEG rapidly evolved due to technological development and digitalization. In 1960s, simultaneous video and EEG recording gave new dimension of EEG. Video EEG currently plays pivotal role in epilepsy diagnosis and presurgical workup. At present EEG is the primary tool to study epileptiform abnormality (interictal and ictal). In parallel with discovery of EEG, there was rapid development in imaging of brain, both structural and functional. With advent of computed tomography (CT) scan followed by magnetic resonance imaging (MRI) and rapid technological advancement in MRI including functional MRI, the understanding of epilepsies has increased many folds. Localization of potential epileptogenic lesion and detection of subtle MRI changes of clinical relevance has led to better surgical outcome. Functional imaging (positron emission tomography and single-photon emission computed tomography) and multimodality imaging have become important tool for clinical and research use.

Despite a substantial progress, investigations in epilepsy has significant unmet needs. The misdiagnosis of epilepsy is as high as 20–30%, mainly because of absence of diagnostic tests, abuse of EEG and other investigations and need for reliable eye-witness account.[13] EEG, the main tool in epilepsy has considerable limitations. It has poor spatial resolution, lacks sensitivity and specificity, and has interobserver variability and lack objectivity. Magnetoencephalography (MEG) is another powerful tools that overcomes some of the drawbacks of EEG.[14] MEG usage is currently limited to few research center, but likely to have more widespread use in future both in clinical and research setting. Till date, we do not have neuroimaging that can detect and differentiate active epileptogenic foci and we rely more on lesion or finding that are abnormal structurally and functionally and can be possible site of seizure origin or cause of epilepsy. The present approach of looking into imaging data along with attempt to correlate it with clinical and EEG data and sometime other ancillary tests helps us to overcome some of current limitations of imaging. However, it needs certain expertize and training and it can lead to error in diagnosis, medical and surgical treatment of epilepsy even at the level of expert. Further improvement in structural and functional neuroimaging might help us to understand epileptogenic area and network of the brain that currently cannot be determined directly.

Other area of future research is to determine reliable biomarker for epilepsy and epileptogenesis and target the process to "cure" epilepsy. Biomarker for epileptogenesis is "an objectively measurable characteristic of a biological process that reliably identifies the development, presence, severity, progression or localization of an epileptogenic abnormality".[15] The development of biomarkers will help in individualizing treatment, prognostication as well as developing strategies to prevent epilepsy by targeting epileptogenesis once potential epileptognic insult has occurred to the brain. The biomarkers that are currently under research are electrophysiological (high-frequency oscillation), genetic, molecular and imaging biomarkers.[16]

TREATMENT OF EPILEPSY: PAST, PRESENT AND FUTURE

Medical Treatment

The introduction of bromide potassium in the treatment of epilepsy by Edward Sieveking in 1857 marked the beginning of modern anti-epileptic treatment. In 1912, Hauptmann (1881-1948), a German physician, discovered anti-epileptic property of phenobarbital while using it as tranquilizer.[1] Phenobarbitone is still widely used and is only anti-epileptic medication available in many resource-poor countries.[17] Search for less-sedative drug led to research and a number of nonsedative phenyl compounds was studied and phenytoin was found to be effective.[18] It was introduced in 1938. Subsequently, primidone, ethosuximide, carbamazepine and valproate were introduced. Benzodiazepines in parallel got established in acute seizure management as well as add-on chronic therapy. Subsequently, there was rapid expansion on AEDs and were termed as "newer" anti-epileptic medications. Many of these molecules had different or novel mechanism of action, giving physician a wider choice of anti-epileptic medications. This expansion of number of AEDs has given opportunity to tailor treatment and helps to minimize the adverse effects. However, despite having newer AEDs, the proportion of medically refractory epilepsy is only marginally change. Almost 30% of epilepsies are poorly controlled despite availability of more than 20 anti-epileptic medications.[19] The increasing understanding of mechanism of drug resistance in epilepsy has also opened the new area of research in form of pharmacogenomics and targeted drug delivery by nanoparticles that may help to overcome some of the mechanism of drug resistance. The incidental observation of dramatic effect of marijuana (cannabinoid) on Dravet's syndrome (a devastating epilepsy syndrome of childhood) has opened a new front of research on anti-epileptic medications with both skepticism and hope.[20]

Medical treatment till date is largely "symptomatic treatment" to control seizure. There is no therapy till date that can alter epileptogenesis. None of the current treatment can prevent development of epilepsy after potential epileptogenic damage to the brain-like stroke, trauma or infections. There are a few promising progress in focal epilepsy as well as epileptogenesis at experimental level. The most widely used vector system for gene therapy in the brain is adeno-associated virus (AAV), which can transfect postmitotic cells (including neurons) with high efficiency and stability and is relatively nonpathogenic.[21]

Looking even further, curing epilepsy may require not only halting epileptogenic processes, but returning synaptic networks to their pre-epileptic state or by creating a compensatory balance to suppress the excess excitability. In order to achieve this target, better understanding of factors in addition to genetic and developmental factors that leads to development of seizure-prone circuits is needed. Why some individuals develop seizures after a given type of brain insult while others do not, remains a subject for future research.

Epilepsy Surgery

There are evidences of trephination of skull was practiced in ancient civilization including India for neurological disorder.[22] However, enthusiasm of surgical treatment for epilepsy started in 19th century and in 20th century, there was rapid development in field of surgical epileptology.[1] Dandy (1886-1946) introduced hemispherectomy as a neurosurgical procedure in 1923. The idea of by surgical removal of abnormal discharging area of brain was put forward by Gibbs and Lennox in 1938. Wilder Penfield (1891-1976) along with Herbert Jasper (1906-1999) and Theodore Brown Rasmussen (1910-2002) in the Neurologic Center of University of Montreal also contributed importantly to the evolution of the surgery of epilepsy. In 1954, Penfield published with Jasper one of the greatest classics in neurology, Epilepsy and the Functional Anatomy of the Human Brain.[23] In 1953, Falconer, a neurosurgeon from New Zealand, introduced anterior temporal lobe resection for temporal lobe epilepsy. In later half of 20th century, epilepsy surgery was practiced at many centers, but encountered lot of skepticism. By the turn of century, Class I evidence for effectiveness of surgery in temporal lobe epilepsy was established[24] and at present plays a very important role in medically refractory epilepsy.

In India, first epilepsy surgery in India was performed on August 25, 1952, by Dr Jacob Chandy at the Christian Medical College (CMC) in Vellore. After initial enthusiasm, there was decline in epilepsy surgery in India. The credit of resurgence of epilepsy surgery in India goes to Professor Kurupath Radhakrishnan, who established India's first dedicated and comprehensive epilepsy center in India in 1994. R Madhavan Nair Comprehensive Epilepsy Center (RMNC), at Sree Chitra Tirunal Institute of Medical Sciences and Technology (SCTIMST), Thiruvananthapuram, Kerala, became the premier center for surgical treatment of epilepsy as well as epilepsy training.[25] The first epilepsy surgery (left anterior temporal lobectomy with amygdalohippocampectomy) at RMNC was conducted on March 20, 1995. Since then, more than 2,000 epilepsy surgeries have been conducted at this center. Epilepsy surgery and centers in steadily growing and average of 420 epilepsy surgery per year is conducted in India.[26] However, there is still huge surgical treatment gap in India.

In future, the epilepsy surgery is likely to become more acceptable, less invasive and safer due to better presurgical localization and planning, delineation of functional areas of brain, improved surgical and postsurgical management. Minimally invasive method, like gamma knife surgery, endoscopic surgery and radiofrequency and thermal ablation method, is likely to play significant role and evolve further with technological refinement.

EPILEPSY AND SOCIETY

The discrimination against epilepsy emerged with belief of supernatural cause that prevails in all civilizations for century. These patients were seen as possessed by devil or demons and seen as cursed by God. This misconception was so deep rooted and prevalent worldwide, that even in 21st century, has significant influence on how society looks toward person with epilepsy (PWE). In India, stigma and taboo are highly prevalent in rural and tribal areas. Even in urban India, it is considerable, but there is steady improvement in social perception and acceptance of PWE in mainstream. Stigma related to epilepsy can lead to underutilization of medical facilities and modern treatment and can defeat the purpose of scientific development.[27] There can be unnecessary restriction including restriction on education by parents or school, unemployment or underemployment leading to long-lasting social, psychological and financial consequences. There is inadequate law to protect rights of PWE in our country. The drive for better legal protection to PWE needs to be intensified. One successful example is abolition of the

Hindu Marriage Act of 1955 and the Special Marriage Act of 1954 that stated that epilepsy at time of marriage can be ground for divorce. It took a struggle of 12 years for the Indian Epilepsy Association to have the word "epilepsy" deleted from this law. This was achieved in December 1999.[28]

The advancement in understanding and therapeutics alone is not enough to fight against epilepsy. We need to empower PWE with knowledge and arm them with law and legislation to protect their right and provide equal opportunity to achieve and perform to their capabilities. On the other hand, education and awareness at community level are necessary to give equal space to PWE.

CONCLUSION

Significant progress has been made in understanding the cause and mechanism of various epilepsies. The therapeutic armamentarium has rapidly expanded in last three decades, but we are still far away from the ideal treatment. The future prospects and upcoming development in pipeline are very promising and there are reasons to hope that epilepsy management in future will be significantly better and have new dimensions like antiepileptogenesis. Due to space limitations, all developments could not be discussed. Finally, the long social injustice to epilepsy needs to be eliminated from society to reap the benefit of rapidly improving scientific development in field of epileptology.

REFERENCES

1. Magiorkinis E, Diamantis A, Sidiropoulou K, Panteliadis C. Highights in the history of epilepsy: the last 200 years. Epilepsy Res Treat. 2014;2014:582039.
2. Jain S, Tandon PN. Ayurvedic medicine and Indian literature on epilepsy. Neurol Asia. 2004;9:57-8.
3. Sidiropoulou K, Diamantis A, Magiorkinis E. Hallmarks in 18th- and 19th-century epilepsy research. Epilepsy Behav. 2010;18:151-61.
4. Gowers WR. The border-land of epilepsy. Faints, vagal attacks, vertigo, migraine, sleep symptoms, and their treatment. Philadelphia: P Blakiston's son & Co; 1903.
5. Jasper H, Kershmann J. Electroencepahlografic classification of the epilepsies. Arch Neur Psych. 1941;45:903-43.
6. Goddard GV. Development of epileptic seizures through brain stimulation at low intensity. Nature. 1967;214:1020-1.
7. Gastaut H. Clinical and Electroencephalographical Classification of Epileptic Seizures. Epilepsia. 1970;11:102-12.
8. Berg AT, Berkovic SF, Brodie MJ, Buchhalter J, Cross JH, Van Emde Boas W, et al. Revised terminology and concepts for organization of seizures and epilepsies: Report of the ILAE Commission on Classification and Terminology, 2005-2009. Epilepsia. 2010;51:676-85.
9. Tedrus GM, Fonseca LC, Melo EM, Ximenes VL. Educational problems related to quantitative EEG changes in benign childhood epilepsy with centrotemporal spikes. Epilepsy Behav. 2009;15:486-90.

10. Jacobsa MP, Leblanca GG, Brooks-Kayalb A, Jensenc FE, Lowensteind DH, Noebelse JL, et al. Curing epilepsy: Progress and future directions. Epilepsy Behav. 2009;14:438-45.
11. Gibbs FA, Gibbs EL, Lennox WG. Epilepsy: a paroxysmal cerebral dysrhythmia. Brain. 1937;60:377-88.
12. Gibbs FA, Gibbs E. Atlas of Electroencephalography. Oxford, UK: Boston City Hospital; 1941.
13. Ferrie CD. Preventing misdiagnosis of epilepsy. Arch Dis Child. 2006;91:206-9.
14. Knowlton RC, Shih J. Magnetoencephalography in epilepsy. Epilepsia. 2004;45:61-71.
15. Engel J Jr. Biomarkers in epilepsy. Biomarkers Med. 2011;5:529-664.
16. Pitkänen A, Löscher W, Vezzani A, Becker AJ, Simonato M, Lukasiuk K. Advances in the development of biomarkers for epilepsy. Lancet Neurol. 2016;15:843-56.
17. Kwan P, Brodie MJ. Phenobarbital for the treatment of epilepsy in the 21st century: a critical review. Epilepsia. 2004;45:1141-9.
18. Merrit H, Putnam T. Sodium diphenyl hydantoinate in the treatment of convulsive disorders. JAMA. 1938;111:1068-73.
19. Sirven JI, Katherine N, Matthew H, Joseph D. Antiepileptic drugs 2012: Recent advances and trends. Mayo Clin Proc. 2012;87:879-89.
20. Rosenberg EC, Tsien RW, Whalley BJ, Devinsky O. Cannabinoids and epilepsy. Neurotherapeutics. 2015;12:747-68.
21. Noè F, Vaghi V, Balducci C, Fitzsimons H, Bland R, Zardoni D, et al. Anticonvulsant effects and behavioural outcomes of rAAV serotype 1 vector-mediated neuropeptide Y overexpression in rat hippocampus. Gene Ther. 2010;17:643-52.
22. Sankhyan AR, Weber GI. Evidence of surgery in ancient India: Trepanation at Burzahom (Kashmir) over 1000 years ago. Int J Osteoarcheol. 2001;11:375-80.
23. Penfield W, Jasper H. Epilepsy and the Functional Anatomy of the Human Brain. Boston, Mass, USA: Little, Brown; 1954.
24. Wiebe S, Blume WT, Girvin JP, Eliasziw M. Effectiveness and Efficiency of Surgery for Temporal Lobe Epilepsy Study Group. A randomized, controlled trial of surgery for temporal-lobe epilepsy. N Engl J Med. 2001;345:311-8.
25. Radhakrishnan K. Epilepsy surgery in India. Neurol India. 2009;57:4-6.
26. Menon RN, Radhakrishnan K. A survey of epilepsy surgery in India. Seizure. 2015;26:1-4.
27. Thomas SV, Nair A. Confronting the stigma of epilepsy. Ann Indian Acad Neurol. 2011;14: 158-63.
28. D'Souza C. Epilepsy and discrimination in India. Neur Asia. 2004;9:53-4.

CHAPTER 2

Epilepsy Classification: Seizures and Syndromes

Ajith Cherian, Divya KP

INTRODUCTION

Seizure is a transient occurrence of symptoms due to an abnormal excessive or synchronous neuronal brain activity. One is diagnosed to have epilepsy if he/she satisfies any of the following:
- A minimum of two unprovoked (or reflex) seizures occurring 24 or more hours apart
- Single unprovoked (or reflex) seizure and a probability of further seizures being at least 60% over the next 10 years (i.e., risk of seizure recurrence is similar as in statement 1)
- Diagnosis of an epilepsy syndrome.[1]

The International League against Epilepsy (ILAE) has incorporated an operational classification of the types of seizure in 2016. It is to recognize those types of seizure that can have either a focal or generalized onset, to classify a seizure when the onset is unobserved, to include some neglected type of seizures, and to adopt more clarity in nomenclature.[2] The 2016 classification is more clinical and practical and based upon the classification published in 1981.[3]

NEED FOR UPDATION

The need of updating the classification of seizures is to:
- Incorporate terms for those types of seizures that did not fit into any prior classification
- Self-explanatory terms for certain types of seizure
- Provide more clarity to the nonmedical community.

FOCAL VERSUS GENERALIZED

In 2010, ILAE defined focal seizures as those brewing within networks which are limited to one hemisphere.[4] They may be either well localized or widely distributed but still confined to one hemisphere. Focal seizures can also emerge from subcortical structures. Generalized seizures were defined as "originating at some point within, and immediately engaging, bilaterally distributed networks." Classifying a seizure as generalized, however, does not rule out a focal onset. From the perspective of epileptic networks, seizures could arise from thalamo-cortical, neocortical, limbic, and brainstem networks. Although our knowledge regarding the electrophysiology of seizure networks is growing rapidly, it is not yet adequate enough to serve as a basis for seizure classification.[5] Physicians have been aware for long that the so-called generalized seizures, for example, generalized absence with electroencephalogram (EEG) showing generalized spike-waves, do not manifest in all parts of the brain uniformly. The Task Force emphasized the concept of bilateral, rather than generalized involvement, since seizures can be bilateral without involving all the brain networks. The term "focal to bilateral tonic-clonic" was substituted for "secondarily generalized." The term "generalized" was retained for those seizures that are generalized from the outset.

ONSET UNKNOWN

In those tonic-clonic seizures where the onset was unobserved, as it often happens when the patient is sleeping, unattended, or caregivers were too carried away by the external manifestations of the seizure to observe the presence of focal features, there is an option to tentatively term this seizure even in the absence of evidence about its origin. The Task Force has hence allowed classification of such seizure type with the revamped term "onset unknown."

CONSCIOUSNESS AND AWARENESS

The 1981 ILAE classification and the later revision in 2010 opined an elementary distinction between seizures with and without impairment of consciousness.[6] A classification based upon consciousness reflects a prudent approach, as seizures with impaired consciousness need to be tackled uniquely from those with no impairment of consciousness, for example, with respect to allowing swimming or driving in adults. Surrogate markers for consciousness often include measurements of awareness, memory, and responsiveness.[7] The 1981 classification distinctly detailed awareness and responsiveness, for the event but excluded ictal memory. Responsiveness may or may not be affected during a focal seizure. Responsiveness cannot be equated to awareness, since some persons may be immobilized or have motor aphasia, and hence, be unresponsive during a seizure, but may still be able to observe and recall their surroundings. The ILAE commission chose the term "awareness" implying an impairment of consciousness to segregate seizure types.[8] The term "awareness unknown" is available when it cannot be ascertained. The term "dyscognitive" was abandoned. Generalized seizures mostly manifest with impaired awareness. Therefore, the presence or impairment of awareness was not included to subclassify generalized seizures. However, responsiveness and awareness can be partially retained even during some of the generalized seizures, for instance absence seizures with eyelid myoclonias[9] or epilepsy with myoclonic absences.[10]

PRACTICAL APPLICATION OF THE CURRENT CLASSIFICATION

The current classification attempts primarily to determine whether the maiden manifestations of the seizure are focal or generalized (Table 1). The seizure is termed "of unknown onset", if the ictal commencement is missed or obscured. The classification of a particular seizure can stop at any stage. It may be branded as "focal" (or "generalized") seizure, with no other descriptives, or named as "focal motor seizure," "focal sensory seizure," "generalized tonic seizure," or any other combination from the given nomenclature. Subsequent classification is encouraged, but discretionary, and their use may depend upon the practical experience of the physician attempting to classify the seizure.[2]

TABLE 1: Current seizure classification

Focal (aware, impaired awareness, unknown awareness)	Generalized	Unknown onset (aware, impaired awareness, unknown awareness)
Motor • Tonic • Atonic • Myoclonic • Clonic • Epileptic spasms • Hypermotor • Nonmotor	**Motor** • Tonic-clonic • Tonic • Atonic • Myoclonic • Myoclonic-atonic • Clonic • Clonic-tonic-clonic • Epileptic spasms	**Motor** • Tonic-clonic • Tonic • Atonic • Epileptic spasms
Nonmotor • Sensory • Cognitive • Emotional • Autonomic	–	**Non-motor** • Unclassified
Focal to bilateral tonic-clonic	**Absence** • Typical • Atypical • Myoclonic • Eyelid myoclonia	–

Focal seizures are subclassified into those with motor and nonmotor features. If both motor and nonmotor symptoms (sensory/autonomic) are present at the onset of seizure, the motor features will usually dominate, unless nonmotor (e.g., sensory) symptoms are very conspicuous.[11] Focal seizures are often accompanied by myriad manifestations, a key feature of which is reduced awareness or consciousness. Impaired awareness is used as a marker for reduced consciousness. A "focal aware seizure" is equivalent to the 1981 nomenclature of "simple partial seizure," and it indicates that awareness, memory, responsiveness, and consciousness are all preserved. Any marked perturbation of any of the foresaid clinical states causes a focal seizure to be termed as having impaired awareness. One may refer to this seizure type as "focal unaware", but it is important to identify that awareness may only be impaired, rather than totally absent. Therefore, the rubric "focal seizure with impaired awareness" is now accepted which corresponds to the 1981 nomenclature "complex partial seizure". If the state of awareness is unknown, then the focal seizure is classified as being "with unknown awareness."

When a focal seizure manifests with more than one of the classifiers under the focal heading, then the assumption is that the one presenting initially and blatantly will be emphasized, since it mirrors the most important culprit regions or networks involved. If multiple sequential features are noticeable, then it is considered as a propagation pattern within one seizure type. One may avoid the term "nonmotor" for focal sensory, cognitive, emotional, or autonomic seizures. The term "aware" may also be avoided for seizure types such as sensory for which awareness is inferred. Order of terms is not critical, such that "focal aware tonic seizure" is the same as "focal tonic seizure with preserved awareness". Where a word can clearly be assumed, it may be avoided, for instance, "generalized tonic seizure," rather than "generalized motor tonic seizure".

The term "focal to bilateral tonic-clonic" is a special seizure type, equivalent to the earlier term "partial onset with secondary generalization." Focal to bilateral tonic-clonic suggests a sequential spread of a seizure, rather than a unique seizure type, but it is such an important and usual presentation that the separate categorization was persisted with. Other types of focal seizures, like tonic or myoclonic may progress or evolve into bilateral tonic-clonic seizures.[12]

Generalized seizures are subdivided into motor and absence seizures. Further nomenclature is similar to those of the 1981 classification, with addition of myoclonic-atonic seizures, seen in epilepsy with myoclonic-atonic epilepsy (Doose syndrome), clonic-tonic-clonic seizures seen in juvenile myoclonic epilepsy,[13,14] myoclonic absence seen in Tassinari syndrome[10] and absence with eyelid myoclonia seizures seen in the syndrome described by Jeavons.[9]

The term "unknown onset" seizures is used for seizure types where the onset is unknown. A spouse may wake up to partner's first tonic-clonic seizure, which would be termed as a seizure of unknown onset (tonic-clonic subtype).If an ensuing ictus is witnessed with a clear focal onset, then the seizure type would be renamed as "focal to bilateral tonic-clonic seizure." An "unclassified seizure" denotes a seizure with no distinction with regard to its nature of onset, presence of motor or nonmotor symptoms, and lack of details about degree of awareness.[15,16] If any of these descriptives are known, then those should be employed to rename the seizure.

ETIOLOGIES

Classification of the type of seizure can be applied irrespective of the etiology. A tumor-induced seizure may be focal irrespective of the state of awareness. Any seizure can become relentless and refractory, leading to status epilepticus of that particular seizure type.[13,14]

AIDING DATA

These include EEG correlates, lesions identified by neuroimaging, and ancillary work up such as antineuronal antibodies, gene mutations.[17-20]

New Lexicon and Description

Some of the older terms have been discarded or replaced by new terms. Table 2 gives details on the commonly replaced terms. A new term hypermotor has been additionally included to focal motor seizure types and substitutes the old usage "hyperkinetic". The term cognitive has replaced "psychic" and refers to specific cognitive disturbances during the seizure, like dysphasia. "Emotional" is used when a focal nonmotor seizure has emotional manifestations, such as cry, fear, or laughter. Specific seizure types that were previously categorized as generalized seizures now also show up under seizures of focal, generalized, and unknown onset. These include epileptic spasms, clonic, tonic, atonic, and myoclonic seizures. As compared to the 1981 classification, new types of generalized seizures included are absence with eyelid myoclonia, myoclonic-atonic, and clonic-tonic-clonic. Some characteristics during focal seizures, like tonic or clonic, can also be witnessed in generalized seizures.

MAJOR CHANGES FROM THE 1981 SCHEME

- Change from "partial" to "focal"
- Few seizure types can be either focal, generalized, or onset unknown
- Seizures of unknown onset can still be classified

TABLE 2: New lexicon and description

Old term for seizure	New term for seizure
Absence	Generalized absence
Akinetic	Generalized/focal/onset unknown atonic
Astatic	Generalized/focal/onset unknown atonic
Atonic	Generalized/focal/onset unknown atonic
Aura	Focal aware
Clonic	Generalized/focal/onset unknown clonic
Complex partial	Focal with impaired awareness
Convulsion	Focal/generalized/onset unknown motor (tonic-clonic, tonic, clonic), focal to bilateral tonic-clonic, tonic-clonic unknown onset
Dacrystic	Focal (aware or impaired awareness) emotional (dacrystic)
Dialeptic	Focal-impaired awareness
Drop attack	Generalized/focal/onset unknown atonic
Fencer's posture	Focal (aware or impaired awareness) motor (tonic)
Figure-of-4	Focal (aware or impaired awareness) motor (tonic)
Freeze	Focal (aware or impaired awareness) arrest
Gelastic	Focal (aware or impaired awareness) emotional (gelastic)
Grand mal	Generalized tonic-clonic, focal to bilateral tonic-clonic, tonic-clonic unknown onset
Gustatory	Focal (aware or impaired awareness) autonomic (gustatory)
Infantile spasms	Generalized/focal/onset unknown epileptic spasms
Jacksonian	Focal aware motor (Jacksonian)
Limbic	Focal impaired awareness
Major motor	Generalized tonic-clonic, focal to bilateral tonic-clonic
Minor motor	Focal motor, generalized myoclonic
Myoclonic	Generalized myoclonic
Partial	Focal
Psychomotor	Focal with impaired awareness
Rolandic	Focal aware motor
Salaam	Generalized/focal/onset unknown epileptic spasms. Secondarily generalized tonic-clonic. Focal to bilateral tonic-clonic
Simple partial	Focal aware
Supplementary motor	Focal motor tonic
Sylvian	Focal motor
Tonic	Generalized/focal/onset unknown tonic
Tonic-clonic	Generalized tonic-clonic, focal to bilateral tonic-clonic, tonic-clonic of unknown onset
Uncinate	Focal (aware or with impaired awareness) sensory (olfactory)

- The terms dyscognitive, simple partial, complex partial, psychic, and secondarily generalized have been eliminated
- Focal (unihemispheric) tonic, clonic, atonic, myoclonic, and epileptic spasms seizure types are recognized, along with bilateral corresponding seizure types
- Addition of new generalized seizure types: absence with eyelid myoclonia, myoclonic absence, clonic-tonic-clonic, myoclonic-atonic, and epileptic spasms.

CLASSIFICATION OF EPILEPSIES

A framework for classification of the epilepsies has been developed. First step is to identify the seizure subtype/s. The second step is to identify whether it is a focal epilepsy, generalized epilepsy, generalized and focal epilepsy, or "unknown if generalized or focal epilepsy".[21-26] At the third level, try to make an epilepsy syndrome diagnosis. Epilepsy syndromes are determined by a distinctive clinical pattern and EEG features. They may have associated imaging, etiological, prognostic, and treatment implications. Best known examples include juvenile myoclonic epilepsy, and benign epilepsy with centro-temporal spikes. The 1989 classification of epilepsies and epileptic syndromes is elaborated in box 1 which is still quite useful for daily practice.

Box 1: Classification of epilepsies and epileptic syndromes (1989)

1. Localization-related epilepsies and syndromes

1.1 Idiopathic
- Benign childhood epilepsy with centrotemporal spikes
- Childhood epilepsy with occipital paroxysms
- Primary reading epilepsy

1.2 Symptomatic
- Chronic progressive epilepsia partialis continua of childhood (Kojewnikow syndrome)
- Syndromes characterized by seizures with specific modes of precipitation
- Temporal lobe epilepsies
- Frontal lobe epilepsies
- Parietal lobe epilepsies
- Occipital lobe epilepsies

1.3 Cryptogenic

2. Generalized epilepsies and syndromes

2.1 Idiopathic
- Benign neonatal familial convulsions
- Benign neonatal convulsions
- Benign myoclonic epilepsy in infancy
- Childhood absence epilepsy
- Juvenile absence epilepsy
- Juvenile myoclonic epilepsy
- Epilepsy with GTCS on awakening
- Other generalized idiopathic epilepsies not defined above
- Epilepsies with seizures precipitated by specific modes of activation

2.2 Cryptogenic or symptomatic
- West syndrome
- Lennox-Gastaut syndrome
- Epilepsy with myoclonic astatic seizures
- Epilepsy with myoclonic absences

Continued

Continued

2.3 Symptomatic

2.3.1 Nonspecific etiology
- Early myoclonic encephalopathy
- Early infantile epileptic encephalopathy with suppression burst
- Other symptomatic generalized epilepsies not defined above

2.3.2 Specific syndromes
- Diseases in which seizures are a presenting or predominant feature

3. Epilepsies and syndromes undetermined whether focal or generalized

3.1 With both generalized and focal seizures
- Neonatal seizures
- Severe myoclonic epilepsy in infancy
- Epilepsy with continuous spike-waves during slow-wave sleep
- Acquired epileptic aphasia (Landau-Kleffner syndrome)
- Other undetermined epilepsies not defined above

3.2 Without unequivocal generalized or focal features (i.e., sleep-related GTCS; when the electroencephalogram shows both focal and generalized ictal or interictal discharges, and when focal or generalized onset cannot be determined clinically)

4. Special syndromes

4.1 Situation-related seizures
- Febrile convulsions
- Isolated seizures or isolated status epilepticus
- Seizures occurring only when there is an acute metabolic or toxic event (alcohol, drugs, eclampsia, nonketotic hyperglycemia)

GTCS, generalized tonic-clonic seizure.

CONCLUSION

The current ILAE revision is operational and not based on mechanisms of seizure genesis. Classification of seizures and epilepsy is the foundation of management. The ILAE classification system is a dynamic work in progress and has been revised and improved over time. The treatment of epilepsy depends on correct classification. Further discussion and feedback from physicians will determine whether the latest classification on seizures will withstand the test of time.

REFERENCES

1. Fisher RS1, Acevedo C, Arzimanoglou A, Bogacz A, Cross JH, Elger CE, et al. ILAE Official Report: A practical clinical definition of epilepsy. Epilepsia. 2014;55(4):475-82.
2. Scheffer IE, French J, Hirsch E, et al. Classification of the epilepsies: New concepts for discussion and debate—Special report of the ILAE Classification Task Force of the Commission for Classification and Terminology. Epilepsia Open. 2016;1–8.
3. Proposal for revised clinical and electroencephalographic classification of epileptic seizures. From the Commission on Classification and Terminology of the International League Against Epilepsy. Epilepsia 1981;22:489.
4. Berg AT1, Berkovic SF, Brodie MJ, Buchhalter J, Cross JH, van Emde Boas W, et al. Revised terminology and concepts for organization of seizures and epilepsies: report

of the ILAE Commission on Classification and Terminology, 2005-2009. Epilepsia. 2010;51:676-85.
5. Blumenfeld H. What is a seizure network? Long-range network consequences of focal seizures. Adv Exp Med Biol. 2014;813:63-70.
6. Blumenfeld H. Impaired consciousness in epilepsy. Lancet Neurol. 2012;11:814-26.
7. Cavanna AE, Monaco F. Brain mechanisms of altered conscious states during epileptic seizures. Nat Rev Neurol. 2009;5:267-76.
8. Shorvon SD. The etiologic classification of epilepsy. Epilepsia. 2011;52:1052-7.
9. Menon R, Baheti NN, Cherian A, Iyer RS. Oxcarbazepine induced worsening of seizures in Jeavons syndrome: Lessons learnt from an interesting presentation. Neurol India. 2011;59:70-2.
10. Cherian A, Jabeen SA, Kandadai RM, Iype T, Moturi P, Reddy M, et al. Epilepsy with myoclonic absences in siblings. Brain Dev. 2014 Nov;36(10):892-8.
11. Rudzinski LA, Shih JJ. The Classification Of Seizures and Epilepsy Syndromes Continuum Lifelong Learning Neurol. 2010;16(3):15-35.
12. Chee MW, Kotagal P, Van Ness PC, Gragg L, Murphy D, Lüders HO, et al. Lateralizing signs in intractable partialepilepsy: blinded multiple-observer analysis. Neurology. 1993;43(12):2519-25.
13. Commission on Classification and Terminology of the International League Against Epilepsy. Proposal for revised classification of epilepsies and epileptic syndromes. Commission on Classification and Terminology of the International League Against Epilepsy. Epilepsia. 1989;30(4):389-99.
14. Engel J Jr; International League Against Epilepsy (ILAE). A proposed diagnostic scheme for people with epileptic seizures and with epilepsy: report of the ILAE Task Force on Classification and Terminology. Epilepsia. 2001;42(6):796-803.
15. Maillard L, Vignal JP, Gavaret M, et al. Semiologic and electrophysiologic correlationsin temporal lobe seizure subtypes. Epilepsia 2004;45(12):1590-9.
16. Bancaud J, Talairach J. Clinical semiology of frontal lobe seizures. AdvNeurol. 1992;57:3-58.
17. Oldani A, Zucconi M, Asselta R, Modugno M, Bonati MT, Dalprà L, et al. Autosomal dominant nocturnal frontal lobeepilepsy: a video-polysomnographic and genetic appraisal of 40 patients anddelineation of the epileptic syndrome. Brain. 1998 Feb;121 (Pt 2):205-23.
18. Ottman R, Winawer MR, Kalachikov S, Barker-Cummings C, Gilliam TC, Pedley TA, et al. LGI1 mutation in autosomal dominantpartial epilepsy with auditory features. Neurology. 2004;62(7):1120-6.
19. Michelucci R1, Poza JJ, Sofia V, de Feo MR, Binelli S, Bisulli F, et al. Autosomal dominant lateral temporal epilepsy: clinical spectrum, new epitempin mutations, and genetic heterogeneity in seven European families. Epilepsia. 2003;44(10):1289-97.
20. Hirose S, Mitsudome A, Okada M, Kaneko S. Genetics of idiopathic epilepsies. Epilepsia 2005;46(suppl 1):38-43.
21. Quesney LF. Clinical and EEG features of complex partial seizures of temporal lobeorigin. Epilepsia 1986;27(suppl 2):S27-45.
22. Michelucci R, Pasini E, Nobile C. Lateral temporal lobe epilepsies: clinical and genetic features. Epilepsia. 2009;50(suppl 5):52-4.
23. French JA, Williamson PD, Thadani VM, et al. Characteristics of medial temporallobe epilepsy: I. results of history and physical examination. Ann Neurol1993;34(6):774–780.
24. Beghi M, Beghi E, Cornaggia CM, Gobbi G. Idiopathic generalized epilepsies of adolescence. Epilepsia. 2006:47(suppl 2):107-10.
25. Xue LY, Ritaccio AL. Reflex seizures and reflex epilepsy. Am J Electroneurodiagnostic Technol. 2006;46(1):39-48.
26. Lüders H1, Acharya J, Baumgartner C, Benbadis S, Bleasel A, Burgess R, et al. Semiological seizure classification. Epilepsia. 1998;39(9):1006-13.

CHAPTER 3

Epilepsy Mimics

Suvasini Sharma, Harsh Patel

INTRODUCTION

The sudden episodic neurologic dysfunction in the form of either altered consciousness or involuntary motor activity or both characterize paroxysmal disorders which pose often diagnostic challenge due to wider differentials.[1] It is noteworthy that everything that twitches or jerks is not a seizure and similarly, not every event associated with loss of consciousness is a seizure. Nonepileptic events can be due to behavioral or psychiatric disturbances, physiological or exaggerated physiological responses, parasomnias, movement disorders, and metabolic or genetic changes.[2] As these are commonly confused with seizures, misdiagnosis of epilepsy is common. Epilepsy mimics can present like epilepsy and may be managed wrongly as epilepsy even for years. There are several conditions closely relating to epilepsy but they are distinct from epilepsy, for example, migralepsy and parasomnia: considered as are at the borderland of epilepsy. Many studies have shown that misdiagnosis rate of epilepsy is as good as 20–30%.[3] This percentage is almost consistent across centers and countries. Epilepsy misdiagnosed pose a significant economic burden to the health system of any nation.[4] On the top of that when a wrong diagnosis of epilepsy has been given, it is easily accepted and perpetuated without being questioned, which explains the diagnostic delay and inappropriate treatment with anti-epileptic drugs (AEDs). In this chapter, common and relevant paroxysmal nonepileptic events that occur in children and may be confused with seizures are discussed. Common seizure mimics in children include breath holding spells, syncope, psychogenic nonepileptic seizures, movement disorders, parasomnias, and physiological events such as sleep myoclonus. Some others that are not so common include shuddering attacks, self-gratification behavior and hyperekplexia.

HOW TO APPROACH

The diagnosing physician is rarely fortunate enough to witnesses the paroxysmal event. It is important to obtain the description of the event from the observer as the information easily becomes distorted if transferred from the observer to the second person and then to physician. Most events are not seizures, and epilepsy should not be a diagnosis of exclusion.[5] Observation of the spell is critical to diagnosis so they hardly remain unexplained when viewed. It is always a good practice to ask the family for recording of the spell. Detailed history regarding the event, just prior to onset, during the event and immediate post event is very vital. Unusual high frequency (multiple daily episodes), refractoriness to AED, unusual triggers like pain, stress, etc. are the red flags against diagnosis of epilepsy.[6] Thoughtful and rational approach to investigations is imperative for correct diagnosis. Electroencephalogram (EEG), video-EEG with recording of event, neuroimaging, and autonomic function tests are useful in appropriate scenario.

PSYCHOGENIC NONEPILEPTIC SEIZURES

Psychogenic nonepileptic seizures (PNES), earlier called as pseudoseizures are episodic, behavioral events that are frequently mistaken for true epileptic seizures. Strictly speaking, terms such as pseudoseizures and nonepileptic seizures include both psychogenic and nonpsychogenic (i.e., organic) epilepsy mimics. A term such as PNES should be preferred because it adds the important connotation of a psychological origin. Lastly, the word seizures are confusing to patients, and for those reasons, psychogenic nonepileptic attacks should be used. They are the most common cause of misdiagnosis of epilepsy.[7] They usually occur due an underlying psychological stressor or conflict. Common stressors include exams, bullying at school, change of school, a new baby in the family, poor school performance, parental discord and rarely, sexual abuse.

In younger children, PNES more commonly present as subtle motor activity such as eye fluttering, isolated head shaking, prolonged staring with unresponsiveness, generalized limpness and behavioral changes such as combativeness.[8] In older children and adolescents, the clinical features are characterized by more prominent motor activity with generalized arrhythmic jerking or flailing of extremities, side-to-side head movements and forward pelvic thrusting.[8] Clinical features which help to differentiate from epilepsy include bizarre semiological features, the fact that these events always occur when awake, in presence of others, apparent resistance to AEDs, and the presence of specific stressful triggers. Sometime patients with true epilepsy may have additional PNES. In these patients, a careful history of the event is helpful to differentiate the semiology of the true seizure versus the PNES.

For the diagnosis, other than the history, review of home videos of the event is helpful. Commonly, it may be possible to try and induce the event in the clinic by means of suggestion. A video-EEG is the gold standard for differentiating true seizures from PNES but this is expensive and usually only reserved for those children in which there is diagnostic confusion between the two. Trials of anti-epileptic medication should not be used to make the distinction. For treatment, the child and family should be referred to a psychologist for evaluation and treatment of the underlying psychopathology.

BREATH-HOLDING SPELLS

Typical breath holding spells usually begin between 6 months and 18 months of age. The child cries in response to anger, frustration, or minor trauma, with sudden cessation of breathing, often during expiration.[5] The child develops cyanosis followed by loss of consciousness and limpness. Loss of tone usually occurs, but in some children tonic posturing and even clonic seizures may appear. Hence, there may be a diagnostic confusion with seizures but what is important to elicit is how the event started.

The pallid breath holding spells are reflex anoxic seizures occurring as a result of asystole of reflex origin.[9] The precipitating factor is usually pain, often due to a minor injury to the head. The child may cry, but crying is minimal and immediately followed by loss of consciousness and tone, with pallor. Tonic posturing of the trunk and limbs with opisthotonus may occur alongwith brief clonic jerks of eyes or limbs. Usually, the child recovers consciousness in less than 1 minute. However, in rare cases, true generalized and even prolonged clonic seizures may follow the tonic episodes. Again, the main diagnostic clue is to elicit the inciting event.

No laboratory tests are needed. A home video of the episode may be helpful. EEG is not indicated unless diagnosis is in doubt and epileptic seizures cannot be conclusively ruled out. If performed, it may reveal slowing or suppression of the background and absence of epileptiform discharges. It is important to differentiate breath-holding from seizures to avoid unnecessary treatment with AEDs. The brief convulsive movements seen during breath-holding spells are reflex anoxic seizures and are not epileptic.

Treatment involves reassuring parents that breath-holding spells are a benign and self-limited condition. Breath-holding may be genetically pre-determined and can be associated with iron deficiency and, therefore, iron supplementation is warranted in these children even in the absence of anemia.

SYNCOPE

Syncope is an abrupt, transient, and self-limiting loss of consciousness associated with loss of postural tone, caused by a sudden fall in cerebral perfusion.[10] Syncope is usually preceded by prodromal symptoms such as blurred vision, light-headedness, dizziness, and nausea. The patient becomes pale. Loss of consciousness and posture tone as well as abrupt unprotected falls may occur. Soon after being in a horizontal position, consciousness returns, but before that myoclonic or clonic jerking of limbs may occur. The most frequent cause of syncope in children and adolescents is

TABLE 1: Major clinical features to differentiate between syncope and seizures[10]

Clinical features	Favors Syncope	Favors Seizures
Provoking factors	• Prolonged sitting or standing; rising to upright posture; dehydration • Pain, fright, onset after exercise • Cough, micturition, defecation, hair brushing, stretch, swallowing cold carbonated beverages, etc.	Sleep deprivation, drug withdrawal (e.g., alcohol, benzodiazepines), photic triggers
Prodrome	• Nausea, palpitations, dyspnea • Warm sensation, lightheadedness, graying of vision, hearing becoming distant	If partial onset, symptoms might indicate temporal, frontal, parietal, or occipital focus
Attack	• Pallor; motionless collapse	Tongue biting, head turning, unusual posturing, urinary incontinence, cyanosis
Postdrome	• Loss of consciousness remembered	Confusion, headache, behaviors (before/during attack) not recalled

vasovagal. Triggers include painful injuries in young children, and emotional disturbances and painful stimuli in adolescents. The tilt test has been shown to be the best procedure to confirm diagnosis of vasovagal syncope.

Cardiogenic syncope must be thought of in all cases with syncope. The long QT syndromes may be associated with life-threatening syncopes, which may be hypotonic or convulsive. The mechanism of the syncope is a ventricular tachyarrhythmia, normally torsades de pointes.[9] A history of syncopal attacks precipitated by exercise or occurring during sleep is strongly suggestive of the long QT syndrome. Table 1 highlights the major differences between syncope and seizures.

GRATIFICATION BEHAVIOR

Gratification behavior, earlier known as infantile masturbation, has onset between 3 months and 3 years. The behavior consists of stereotyped episodes of variable duration (minutes to rarely hours) consisting of vocalizations with quiet grunting, facial flushing with diaphoresis, pressure on the perineum with characteristic posturing of the lower extremities (usually adduction). There is no alteration of consciousness. They usually occur when the child is tired, sleepy or bored.

The event can be stopped by distracting the child. These children are otherwise normal. No laboratory studies are indicated. The parents should be reassured.

MOVEMENT DISORDERS

There are a lot of movement disorders such as dystonias, tics, tremors, choreoathetoid movements, and paroxysmal dyskinesias, which can mimic seizures. The diagnosis is usually not difficult once the movements are observed on clinical evaluation or home videos. Movement disorders do not occur in sleep. The paroxysmal dyskinesias are not so common and the disorders characterized by episodic hyperkinetic movements (dystonia, chorea, ballism, or a mixture), which are not associated with impairment of consciousness. Three main subtypes are recognized (Table 2). Clinically, these disorders are closely resemble to focal motor seizures, although they are distinguishable by their reproducible triggers and absence of secondary generalization.[10]

SHUDDERING ATTACKS

Shuddering attacks usually present in infancy at 4-6 months of age, rarely occurring after the age of 3 years. The attacks usually last for a few seconds. They are characterized by rapid shivering of the body with sudden flexion of head, trunk and elbows, adduction of elbows and knees and no alteration of consciousness.[9] This activity is similar to shivering that occurs when exposed to cold. The episodes occur in clusters, several times a day. The pathophysiology is not known. Parents need to be reassured that this is a benign, self-limited condition and no treatment is necessary.

TABLE 2: Overview of main subtypes of paroxysmal dyskinesia[10]

	Triggers	Attack duration and frequency	Onset and progression	Treatment
Paroxysmal non-kinesogenic dyskinesia	Caffeine, alcohol, sleep deprivation, stress	Typically 10 min to 1 hr; usually <1 attack per week	Onset 3 months to 12 years (mean 4 years); improvement in adulthood	Benzo-diazepines, acetazolamide
Paroxysmal kinesogenic dyskinesia	Sudden voluntary movement	<1 min; commonly multiple attacks per day	Onset 1–20 years (mean 11.6 years); improvement or remission common after 20 years of age	Carbamazepine, phenytoin
Paroxysmal exertion-induced dyskinesia	Prolonged exertion (e.g., 15–60 min), fasting, stress	<1 min to 2 hr; frequency variable	Onset: 2–30 years; progression variable	Glucose responsive, ketogenic diet

STEREOTYPIES

Stereotypies are repetitive, simple movements that can be voluntarily suppressed. Motor stereotypies occur commonly but not exclusively in autistic spectrum disorders. Similar movements are also found in otherwise healthy children, especially when they are excited and those suffering sensory impairment, social isolation, or severe intellectual disabilities; they may be persistent over time.[9] The common types include repeated hand flapping and waving. The characteristic feature of these movements is that they cease when the child is distracted. They appear generally when the child is excited, stressed or bored.

PAROXYSMAL NONEPILEPTIC EVENTS IN SLEEP

Paroxysmal nonepileptic events occur predominantly or exclusively in sleep. It is often difficult to distinguish such phenomenon from true seizures. The most common of these are parasomnias. Those that are confused with seizures include nonrapid eye movement (NREM) arousal disorder parasomnias (confusional arousals, sleep terrors and sleep walking) or rapid eye movement (REM) sleep behavior disorders. Confusional arousals are the most common parasomnias, affecting up to 20% of children. They are associated with sudden arousals, disorientation, prolonged confused behavior and slow, and nonsensical speech.[9] Children have no memory of the attacks on waking the following morning. Sleep terrors (night terrors) are typically seen in young children and are characterized by abrupt arousal with loud and inconsolable crying and screaming. The child seems terrified but tends fall asleep again and will not recall the event later. When associated with excessive motor activity such as thrashing of limbs, there can be a diagnostic confusion with frontal lobe seizures which also occur characteristically during sleep. Some characteristics which help to differentiate the two include brief duration of seizures (usually less than 1 minute), seizures being stereotyped (same semiology during each event) and frequent occurrence of dystonic posturing during seizures (Table 3).[7]

TABLE 3: Salient clinical features for frontal lobe seizures and parasomnias[6]

Frontal lobe seizures	Parasomnias
Onset in childhood or adult	Usually in childhood can persist in adulthood
Stereotyped variable	Variable
Short: Up to 1 minute	Longer several minutes
Frequent, e.g., many per night	Infrequent, for example, once per night
Any time in sleep	Early in sleep (NREM parasomnia) late in sleep (REM parasomnia)
No amnesia (often retain awareness)	Amnesia (but may recall dream from REM-sleep behavior disorder)

REM, rapid eye movement; NREM, non-rapid eye movement.

HYPEREKPLEXIA

Hyperekplexia is an inherited disorder characterized by excessive startle reflexes. Clinical hallmarks of this disorder include excessive auditory and tactile startle, continuous stiffness in the neonatal period, and startle-induced falling.[11] They should be differentiated from seizures for prompt recognition and management. Hyperekplexia is most commonly caused by dominant or recessive mutations in the *GLRA1* gene, which encodes the α1 subunit of the glycine receptor.

The onset is at birth or early infancy.[10] When the onset is at birth, the newborn may appear hypotonic during sleep and develop generalized stiffening on awakening. Apnea and an exaggerated startle response are associated signs. Nose tapping test is a useful clinical sign to induce startle reflex in controlled environment. The stiffening response is often confused with the stiff man syndrome. Other findings include periodic limb movements in sleep (PLMS) and hypnagogic (occurring when falling asleep) myoclonus. Intellect is usually normal. A family history of startle disease helps the diagnosis, but often is lacking. In startle disease, unlike startle-provoked epilepsy, the EEG is always normal. Clonazepam is the most effective and valproate and levetiracetam are also useful.

CONCLUSION

Nonepileptic paroxysmal events that mimic seizures are common in children. A good history is a must for appropriate diagnosis—especially the circumstances, description, and what happened after the event. It is helpful to try to witness event by means of home videos. Investigations are seldom helpful. A routine EEG is not helpful in ruling out epilepsy. Video-EEG may be useful in some situations where there is a diagnostic confusion.

REFERENCES

1. Smith PE. The bare essentials: epilepsy. Pract Neurol. 2008;8:195-202.
2. Mackay M. Fits, faints and funny turns in children. Aust Fam Physician. 2005;34(12):1003-8.
3. Benbadis S. The differential diagnosis of epilepsy: a critical review. Epilepsy Behav. 2009;15(1):15-21.
4. Juarez-Garcia A, Stokes T, Shaw B, Camosso-Stefinovic J, Baker R. The costs of epilepsy misdiagnosis in England and Wales. Seizure. 2006;15, 598-605.
5. Fejerman N. Nonepileptic disorders imitating generalized idiopathic epilepsies. Epilepsia. 2005;46(Suppl 9):80-3.
6. Smith PE. Epilepsy: mimics, borderland and chameleons. Pract Neurol. 2012;12(5):299-307.
7. Bodde NM, Brooks JL, Baker GA, Boon PA, Hendriksen JG, Mulder OG, et al. Psychogenic non-epileptic seizures—definition, etiology, treatment and prognostic issues: a critical review. Seizure. 2009;18:543-53.

8. Patel H, Dunn DW, Austin JK, Doss JL, Plioplys S, Caplan R. et al. Psychogenic nonepileptic seizures (pseudoseizures). Pediatr Rev. 2011;32(6):e66-72.
9. Sankhyan N. Non-epileptic paroxysmal events mimicking seizures. Indian J Pediatr. 2014;81(9):898-902.
10. Crompton DE, Berkovic SF. The borderland of epilepsy: clinical and molecular features of phenomena that mimic epileptic seizures. Lancet Neurol. 2009;8(4):370-81.
11. Bakker MJ, van Dijk JG, van den Maagdenberg AM, Tijssen MA. Startle syndromes. Lancet Neurol. 2006;5:513-24.

4
CHAPTER

Epilepsy Diagnosis

Shiva Kumar R

INTRODUCTION

Various studies have shown that a significant proportion of epilepsy diagnosis made by nonspecialists (like general practitioners and physicians) are incorrect leading to physical, psychosocial, and economic implications for the patient along with unwanted investigations and exposure to antiseizure medications.[1-3] Diagnosis of epilepsy is difficult in the early stages, especially, if one does not have eye witness. Diagnosis of epilepsy is even more difficult in children with a learning disability and in elderly with multiple comorbidities.

An epilepsy specialist (epileptologist) has been defined as a trained doctor with expertise in epilepsy as demonstrated by training and continuing education in epilepsy, peer review of practice, and regular audit of diagnosis. Epilepsy must be a significant part of their workload (equivalent to at least one session a week) in their clinical practice.[4]

CLINICAL EVALUATION

One of main goals in the clinical evaluation of a person suffering from epilepsy is to identify the correct seizure type and to identify the correct epilepsy syndrome for appropriate selection of medications and prognosis. Commonly used terms in epilepsy are described in table 1. Recently, the International League Against Epilepsy (ILAE) updated seizure classification[5,6] and is described in detail elsewhere.

Important questions one has to answer during the diagnosis of epilepsy are:
- Are the paroxysmal events epileptic seizures?
- If epileptic, what type of epileptic seizures? Any specific precipitating and predisposing factors?
- What is the epileptic syndrome or epileptic disease?
- What is the cause (etiology)? Is there a treatable underlying cause?
- Disability associated with epilepsy. For example, driving, education, marriage, fertility, etc.

Epilepsy Diagnosis

TABLE 1: Commonly used terms in epilepsy

Term	Definition
Seizure	Seizure is an event caused by abnormal, excessive, and hyper-synchronous discharge from a group of neurons in the brain ("epileptic focus")
Epilepsy syndrome	Epileptic disorder characterized by a cluster of signs and symptoms occurring together, including seizure type, precipitating factors, age of onset, and severity
Drug-resistant epilepsy	Failure of adequate trials of two tolerated, appropriately chosen, and administered (at least 6 months) anticonvulsant drug (whether in monotherapy or in combination) to achieve seizure freedom

CLINICAL HISTORY

Diagnosis of epilepsy is almost always based solely on detailed clinical history. History should be obtained carefully from the patient, family member, and the available eye witnesses. In simple partial seizures, conscious patients can describe most of the details occurring during the seizures. However, if consciousness is impaired, history obtained from the eye witness or the family member is very important.

Sometimes, the diagnosis is easy based on the details provided by the patient or the eye witness. However, in situations, where clinical details are not available or inadequate, one has to enquire for other details like precipitating factors, circumstances leading to attacks, and for associated signs like incontinence, tongue bite, fractures, and joint dislocations. More difficult cases need video-electroencephalography (video-EEG) documentation.[7,8] Recording of events on the mobile phones and camcorders at home has reduced the need for video-EEG monitoring in recent times. Figure 1 shows video-EEG recording in a 34-year-old female presenting with episodes of confusion lasting for a minute without any automatisms, motor and sensory manifestations for about 2 years.

"Reflex seizures" (which are the result of sensory stimulation caused by the environment) are triggered by visual stimuli (flashing lights or rapidly changing or alternating images as in clubs, around emergency vehicles), sunlight, reading, hot water, eating, and music. Figure 2 shows a video-EEG recording in a boy to document jerks noted while playing a game on mobile phone.

A person is considered to have epilepsy, if they meet any of the following conditions:[5]
- At least two unprovoked (or reflex) seizures occurring greater than 24 hours apart
- One unprovoked (or reflex) seizure and a probability of further seizures similar to the general recurrence risk (at least 60%) after two unprovoked seizures, occurring over the next 10 years

Epilepsy

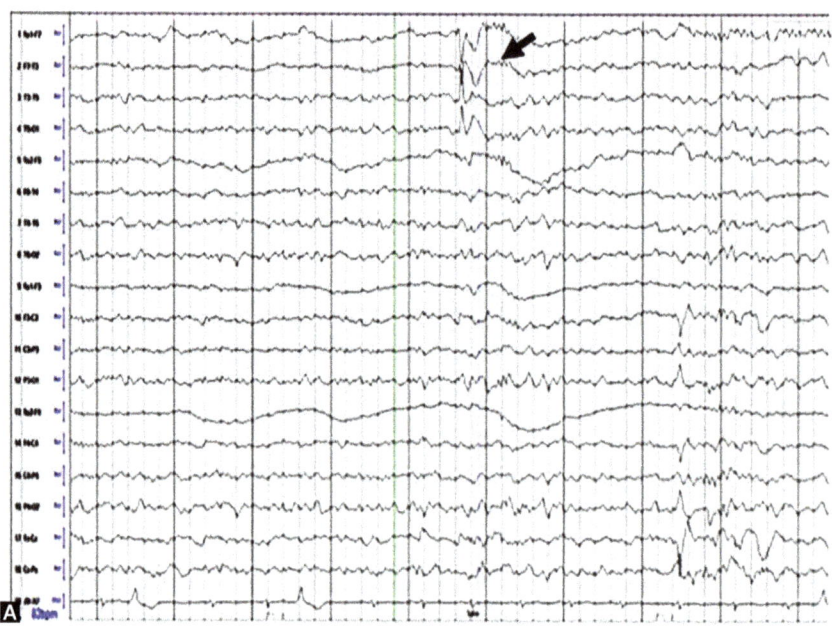

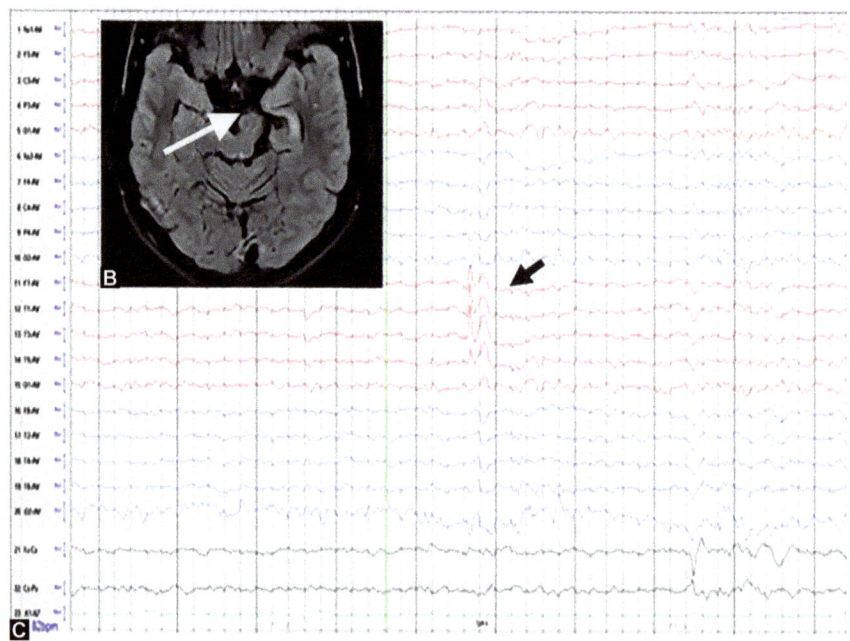

Continued

Continued

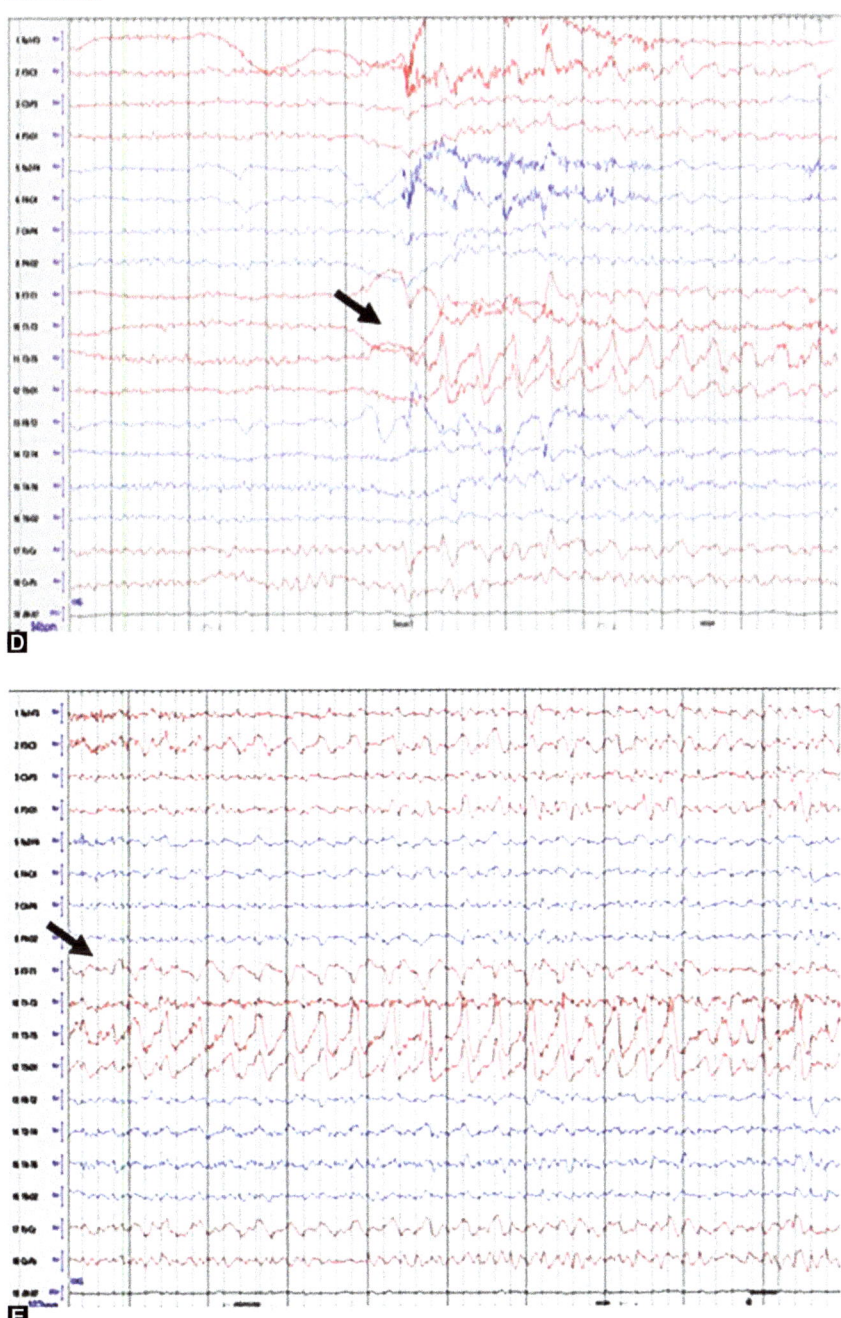

FIG. 1: Video-EEG in a 34-year-old lady with episodic confusion. EEG (**A and C**) showing left temporal sharp wave (pointed arrows). MRI (**B**) axial FLAIR sequence showing left hippocampal volume loss with signal changes (typical of mesial temporal sclerosis). EEG during a seizure (**D**) showing evolving ictal pattern over the left temporal region

Epilepsy

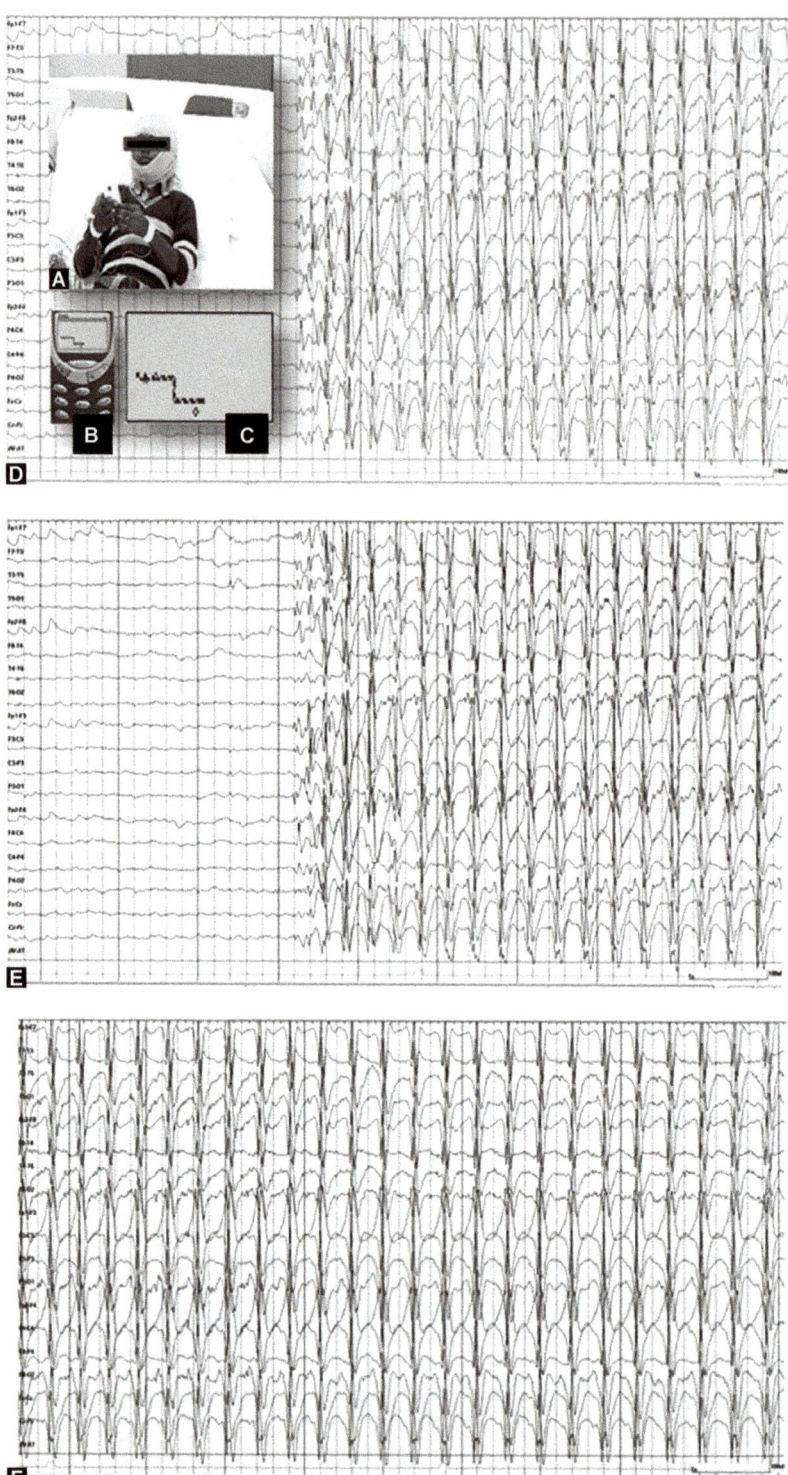

Continued

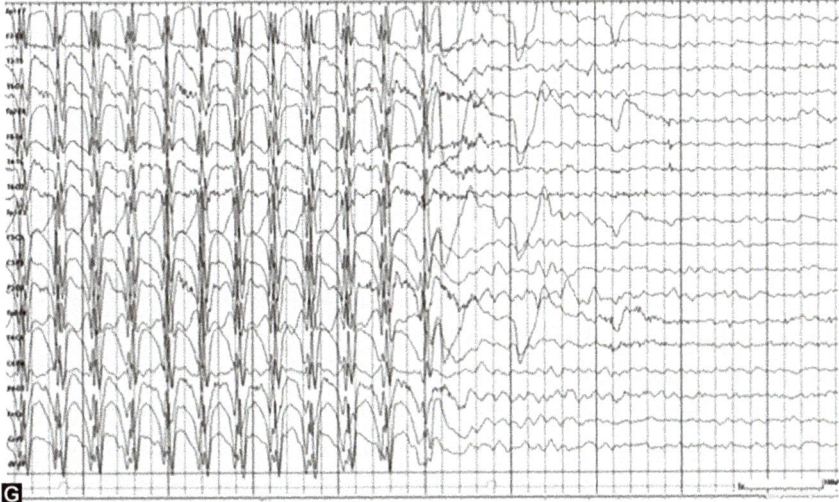

FIG. 2: Video-EEG (**A**) in a boy done to document jerks noted while playing a "snake game" on Nokia mobile phone (**B and C**) showing rhythmic jerks in the neck and limbs. EEG during the jerks (**D, E, F and G**) showing 3 Hz generalized frontally dominant spike and wave discharges

- Diagnosis of an epilepsy syndrome
- Epilepsy is considered to be resolved for individuals who had an age-dependent epilepsy syndrome, but are now past the applicable age or those who have remained seizure-free for the last 10 years with no seizure medicines for the last 5 years.

"That's It!" Phenomenon[9]

At times, it is necessary to ask the eye witness or the family member to imitate and physically demonstrate the events for clarification. Sometimes, it is necessary for the physician or a neurologist to imitate and demonstrate physically or when in doubt, to show video-EEG recorded examples of different epileptic or nonepileptic seizures in order to confirm the paroxysmal event as seizures: the "that's it!" phenomenon.

Description of Seizures: Seizure Semiology

Once we have confirmed that the paroxysmal event is genuinely epileptic, the next step is to define the type of seizure or seizures, which is mandatory for the correct diagnosis and management (Flowchart 1). A detailed description (seizure semiology) of what happens to the patient before a seizure (prodrome and aura), during the seizure (ictus or ictal), and after the seizure (postictal) is very important. Video recording of the events at home will be valuable for correct description of seizure semiology.

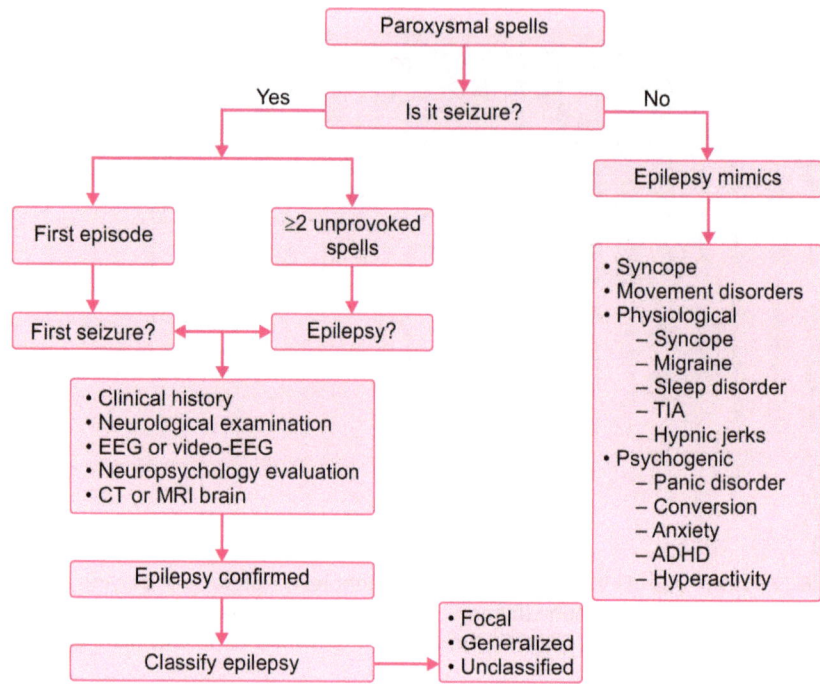

EEG, electroencephalography; CT, computed tomography; MRI, magnetic resonance imaging; TIA, transient ischemic attack; ADHD, attention-deficit hyperactivity disorder.

FLOWCHART 1: Algorithm for epilepsy diagnosis and management

Manifestations of seizures range from the dramatic events of a generalized tonic-clonic seizure (GTCS) to the mild flickering of the eyelids or unawareness or automatisms of the mouth. Minor events also called as small seizures by the patient or family members are often overlooked in the history and are in fact more important than a GTCS in the diagnosis of epilepsies. The same patient may suffer from different types of minor and major seizures, independently or evolving from one to the other.

People with epilepsy are unlikely to report minor seizures because they do not appreciate their significance

Physician's responsibility is to detect minor seizures and evaluate them.

The examiner must note the following details in seizure history:
- Age of onset of first seizures along with detailed description of the first event[10]
    - Age of onset is diagnostically useful as many causes of epilepsy and most specific epilepsy syndromes are age related
- Detailed note of different types of seizures the patient has experienced (for example: in juvenile myoclonic epilepsy presenting with GTCS, a detailed history should be taken to uncover previous myoclonic jerks and absence seizures)[11,12]

- Age of onset, frequency, and evolution of seizures over time should be determined
  - Evolution of symptoms may also suggest progression of the underlying pathophysiological process (for example: enlarging epileptogenic lesion such as neoplasm or degenerative disease)
- Antiseizure drug history:
  - Complete list of all medications tried in the past
  - Highest doses and the length of time each medication tried
  - Efficacy and side effects of each medication
  - Reason for termination of antiseizure medications should also be noted.

Improper use or unnecessary termination of effective drugs is a frequent cause of apparent medical intractability (pseudorefractory epilepsy).

Prodrome

- Presence of prodrome and aura should be determined in every epilepsy patient
- Prodrome is a preictal phenomenon and is not a seizure. Prodrome is a subjective clinical alteration (e.g., ill-localized sensation or agitation) that precedes the onset of an aura and epileptic seizure, but does not form part of it.

Aura

- Aura is a subjective ictal phenomenon that may precede an observable seizure. Rarely auras can occur after seizures (postictal auras)
- Consciousness is preserved during aura and one is aware of the surroundings
- Auras can be in the form of olfactory, visual and auditory hallucination, lightheadedness, Deja vu, abnormal taste, abdominal sensation, and indescribable sensation
- Duration of aura (varies from few seconds to more than 5 minutes) and the consistency with which it precedes the seizure should be noted
- Auras can occur in isolation without any seizure (only auras = simple sensory seizure)
- Often presence of aura indicates that the seizure is focal in origin
- Once recognized as a reliable warning, auras and prodromal symptoms often provide an opportunity for the patient to avoid injury or embarrassment during an epileptic attack.

Ictal Phase

The clinical manifestations during a seizure are known as ictus and have to be described in detail from the onset to the end by a reliable eye witness. The description should include temporal sequence of any arrest of movement, autonomic changes and alteration in consciousness, the part of the body and the side involved in jerks, or tonic or clonic movements. Degree of consistency from one seizure to another is very important in seizure description (stereotypy). Based on clinical manifestations and EEG findings, seizures are classified as focal (also called as partial) and generalized.

Generalized Seizure (Primary or Secondary)

In generalized seizures consciousness is impaired at onset due to simultaneous involvement of both cerebral hemispheres and with bilateral motor manifestations. EEG changes are bilateral at onset and widespread over both hemispheres (Fig. 3). Generalized seizures may be convulsive or nonconvulsive. Generalized seizures may be primary or secondarily generalized. **Primarily** generalized seizures or *idiopathic* are generalized from the onset. **Secondary** generalized seizures are partial (focal) at onset and then spread over both hemispheres triggering a generalized fit.[12,13]

Focal (Partial) Seizure

A seizure is partial when the initial clinical and electrographic manifestations indicate an origin in one cerebral hemisphere (Fig. 4). What happens to the person during the seizure depends on part of the brain involved during a seizure. Depending on impairment of consciousness focal seizures are classified as simple and complex partial seizures.

- Simple partial seizures may manifest with motor signs, somatosensory or special sensory symptoms, autonomic signs or symptoms, or with

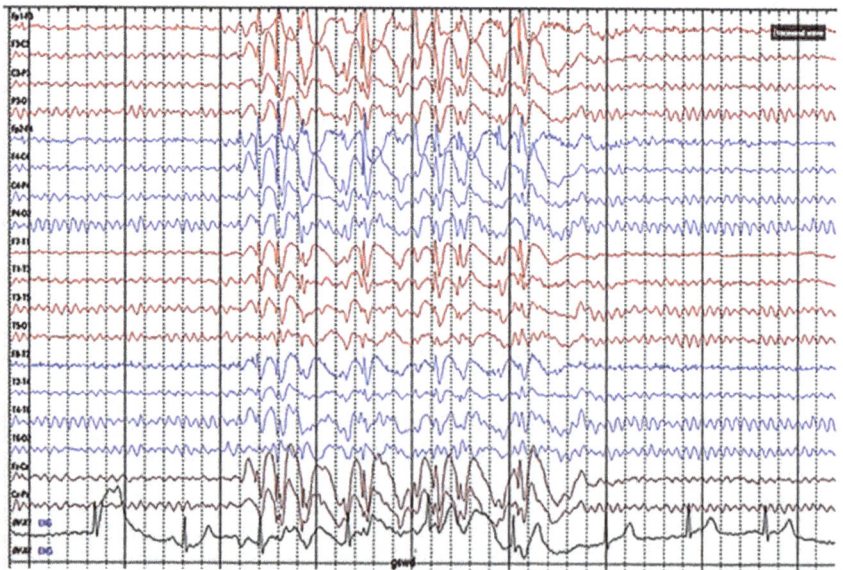

FIG. 3: Electroencephalography of a 10-year-old girl with poor academics showing generalized atypical, fast frontally dominant 3.5–4 Hz spike, and wave discharges suggestive of primary generalized epilepsy

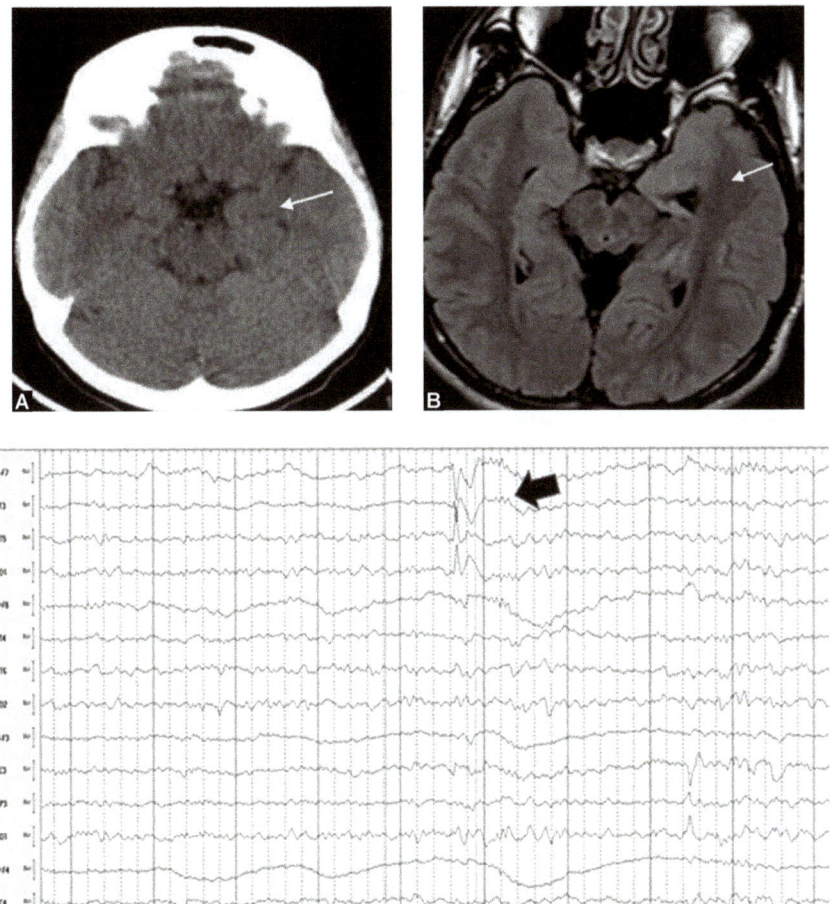

FIG. 4: A 25 year old girl with febrile seizures in childhood and medically refractory focal (complex partial seizures) epilepsy. **A,** Computed tomography scan. brain normal. **B,** Magnetic resonance imaging brain shows hyperintense signals in the left amygdala, uncus, and hippocampus with atrophy and dilated temporal horn (hippocampal sclerosis) classical of mesial temporal sclerosis (arrow). **C,** Electroencephalography show left temporal sharp waves (arrow)

psychic symptoms. Somatosensory or special sensory symptoms vary depending on the region of cortical involvement and are generally positive phenomenon. Primary somatosensory seizures are felt as tingling or as pins or needles sensations and can spread (Jacksonian march) along regions subserved by the sensory homunculus. Autonomic activity may in the form of goose bumps, flushing, pallor, sweating, and change in heart rate, breathing, and blood pressure.

A Jacksonian seizure is a type of simple focal motor seizure characterized by abnormal movements that begin in one group of distal muscles and progress to adjacent groups of muscles. If these focal motor seizures are unremitting then they are called as epilepsia partialis continua.

Impaired consciousness is defined as the inability to respond normally to external stimuli by virtue of altered awareness and/or responsiveness. Complex partial seizures can evolve either from simple partial seizures or they can begin with impaired consciousness *de novo*. Simple partial seizures that begin at onset are considered as auras and they are generally forgotten as a part of perictal amnesia.

Complex partial seizures can be further classified into seizures with and without automatisms. Automatisms are complex release behaviors that emerge with impairment of consciousness. Automatisms are learned behaviors and can manifest in the form of chewing, speaking, gesturing, walking, or making facial expressions.

Postictal Phase

Following a seizure, the person enters into the postictal state. Various postictal phenomenons are frequently noted and include fatigue, drowsiness, headache, confusional state, Todd's paresis, and psychosis. Duration of postictal period may vary from few minutes to days and should not be confused with ictal duration, which rarely lasts for more than 40-60 seconds in generalized seizure and a minute or two in complex partial seizures.

Todd's paresis (Todd's palsy) is focal weakness in a part of the body and typically affects appendages. It usually subsides completely within 48 hours. Todd's paresis may also affect speech, eye position (gaze), or vision. Postictal psychosis and aphasia have lateralizing value in diagnosis of epilepsy.

Other History in Diagnosis of Epilepsy

- Circumstances under which seizures have occurred:
    - Timing of seizures (circadian distribution—nocturnal, on awakening or diurnal)
    - Standing or sitting (helps to differentiate from epilepsy mimics like syncope)
    - At rest or during exercise
    - Possible triggering, precipitating, or facilitating factors (has implications in treatment):
        - Watching television and playing video games (Fig. 2)
        - Exposure to sunlight and flickering lights
        - Sleep deprivation and working in shifts
        - Stress, febrile illness, and fasting during festivals

Epilepsy Diagnosis

- – Missing medications
  - Frequency of seizures:
    - – Seizure diary helps in knowing frequency of each type of seizure and assessing epilepsy disability and effectiveness of therapy
- Past medical history—provides clues to etiology:
  - Complications during gestation, birth trauma, postictal intracranial infections, and serious head injury are common causes of epilepsy
  - Febrile seizures or febrile status lasting for more than 30 minutes
  - Development history in children to differentiate between progressive degenerative neurological disorder and a static lesion
  - Medications history
- Social history:
  - Level of education, occupation, and living arrangements
  - Marital status and use of contraceptives
  - Driving
  - Nicotine, caffeine, alcohol, and recreational drug use
- Family history:
  - History of febrile seizures and epilepsy in family (genetic epilepsy with febrile seizure plus)
  - Left handedness in the absence of a family history of sinistrals and raises suspicion of early injury to the left cerebral hemisphere
- Epilepsy related comorbidities:
  - Headache (migraine); depression, suicidal ideations; quality of life in epilepsy (QOLIE)
  - In children-learning disabilities, anxiety, and attention deficit hyperactivity disorder.

GENERAL PHYSICAL EXAMINATION

Detailed general examination helps in finding specific physical signs or malformations that cause epileptic seizures. Evidence for systemic side effects of antiseizure medications may also be noted during examination. For example, phenytoin can cause coarse facial features, hirsutism, gingival hyperplasia, and rickets in children. Simple bedside hyperventilation can trigger absence seizures in children.

- Vital parameters like heart rate, blood pressure, and detailed cardiac examination may help to differentiate convulsive syncope from epileptic seizures
- Dermatological abnormalities—axillary freckling, nevus anemicus and café au lait spots associated with neurofibromatosis; Port Wine stain of Sturge-Weber syndrome; ash-leaf spots, facial sebaceous adenoma, and shagreen patch of tuberous sclerosis
- Funduscopic examination helps to look for retinal abnormalities that may be seen in association with brain malformations or storage disorders

- Dysmorphic facial and body features provide clues to presence of brain malformations
- Head circumference for micro- or macrocephaly in infants and children
- Auscultation of the head for bruits for vascular malformations
- Abdominal examination for hepatosplenomegaly seen in children with storage disorders.

NEUROLOGICAL EXAMINATION

Neurological examination is often normal in patients with epilepsy. Abnormal neurological findings suggest either diffuse or focal structural or metabolic abnormalities and provide useful localizing and lateralizing information. Specific motor and sensory deficits can be seen with disturbances in the primary cortical regions. Visual field defects indicate lesion in the posterior cortex (posterior temporal and parieto-occipital region).

INVESTIGATION IN THE DIAGNOSIS OF EPILEPSY

Electroencephalography

- Electroencephalography remains the sinlge most noninvasive test in the diagnosis of epilepsy and is often misused
- Overinterpretation of EEG is the most common cause of unwarranted diagnosis of epilepsy
- Unnecessary EEG procedures result in unavoidable expense and inconvenience
- Electroencephalography is not a substitute for good history. But can add value to the diagnosis of epilepsy
- An EEG should be obtained in all patients with epilepsy to provide baseline data that can be used if clinical picture changes
- Electroencephalography can be of help to:
  - Confirm the diagnosis of epilepsy
  - Classify the type of epilepsy and epilepsy syndrome
  - Localization of epilepsy
  - Effectiveness of treatment in epilepsy
  - Predicting the risk of recurrence after first seizure
- Yield of EEG is higher if done within 48 hours of the seizure or epilepsy.[14]

"Normal EEG does not rule out the possibility of epilepsy"

Video-electroencephalography Monitoring in Diagnosis and Classification

- Video-EEG monitoring refers to continuous EEG recorded for a prolonged period with simultaneous video recording of the clinical manifestations

Epilepsy Diagnosis

- Having a correlation of the recorded behavior (video) and the EEG activity, the diagnosis of seizures or nonepileptic seizures can be made definitely in nearly all cases
- Video-EEG helps to classify seizure types, assess seizure frequency, identifies seizure triggers, and localize seizure onset in refractory focal epilepsies
- Additional physiologic parameters like electrocardiogram, heart rate, electrooculogram, electromyogram, and respiratory function can be monitored, which helps in differentiating physiologic nonepileptic disorder associated with paroxysmal clinical events
- Video-EEG monitoring is essential in determining the localization of the epileptogenic zone (i.e., the site of seizure onset and initial seizure propagation) in adult patients being considered for surgical-ablative procedures.[14]

"When clinical information and standard investigations do not allow a confident diagnosis, referral for the recording of attacks should be considered."

Ambulatory Electroencephalography

- 24–72 hours of EEG recorded in a special recorder worn over the wrist
- During the test, one has to keep a diary of what you do during the day and if you have had any seizures or other symptoms.

Neuropsychological Tests

- To evaluate memory and language functions and help to lateralize to right or left hemisphere
- Help lateralization and localization of areas of brain that are abnormal
- Baseline assessment before like epilepsy surgery for its risk on memory and cognition.

Neuroimaging in Epilepsy[15]

Imaging of brain is indicated in almost all patients suspected of having seizures and aid in syndromic and etiological diagnosis. Scans must be interpreted in the context of entire clinical situation. A specialist in neuroimaging, who has training and expertise in the neuroimaging of epilepsy, must review the images.

- Computed tomography (CT) scan brain—can only detect gross lesions and calcifications
- Magnetic resonance imaging (MRI) brain (ideally 1.5 Tesla and 3 Tesla)— imaging modality of choice:
  - Superior to CT scan in identifying lesional epilepsies (hippocampal sclerosis, malformations of cortical development, vascular malformations, tumors, granulomas, trauma and strokes) (Figs 5 and 6)

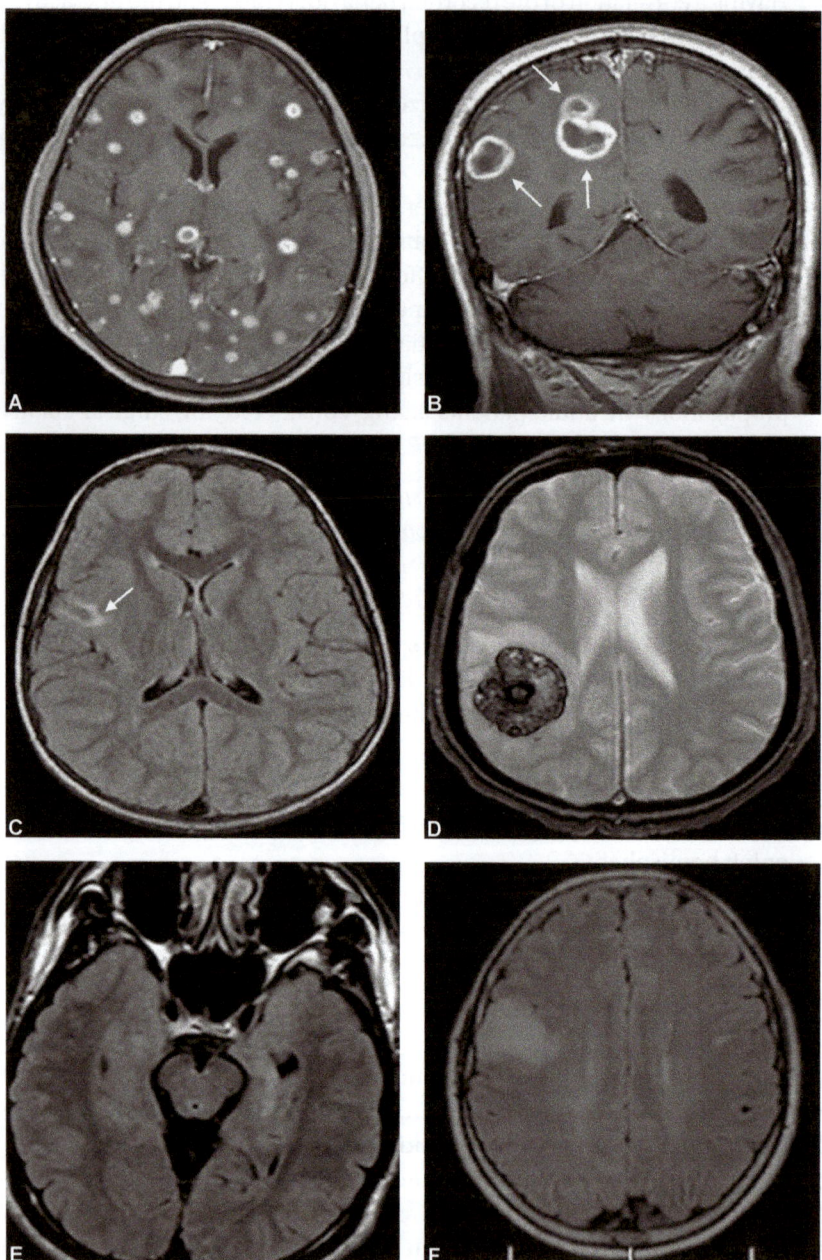

FIG. 5: A, Magnetic resonance imaging (MRI) contrast showing ring enhancing lesions (cysticercosis); **B,** MRI contrast showing ring enhancing lesions (tuberculomas); **C,** MRI showing malformations of cortical development (dysplasia); **D,** MRI showing right frontal cavernoma; **E,** MRI showing volume loss and left hippocampal hyperintensity; **F,** MRI showing focal cortical dysplasia in the right frontal

Epilepsy Diagnosis

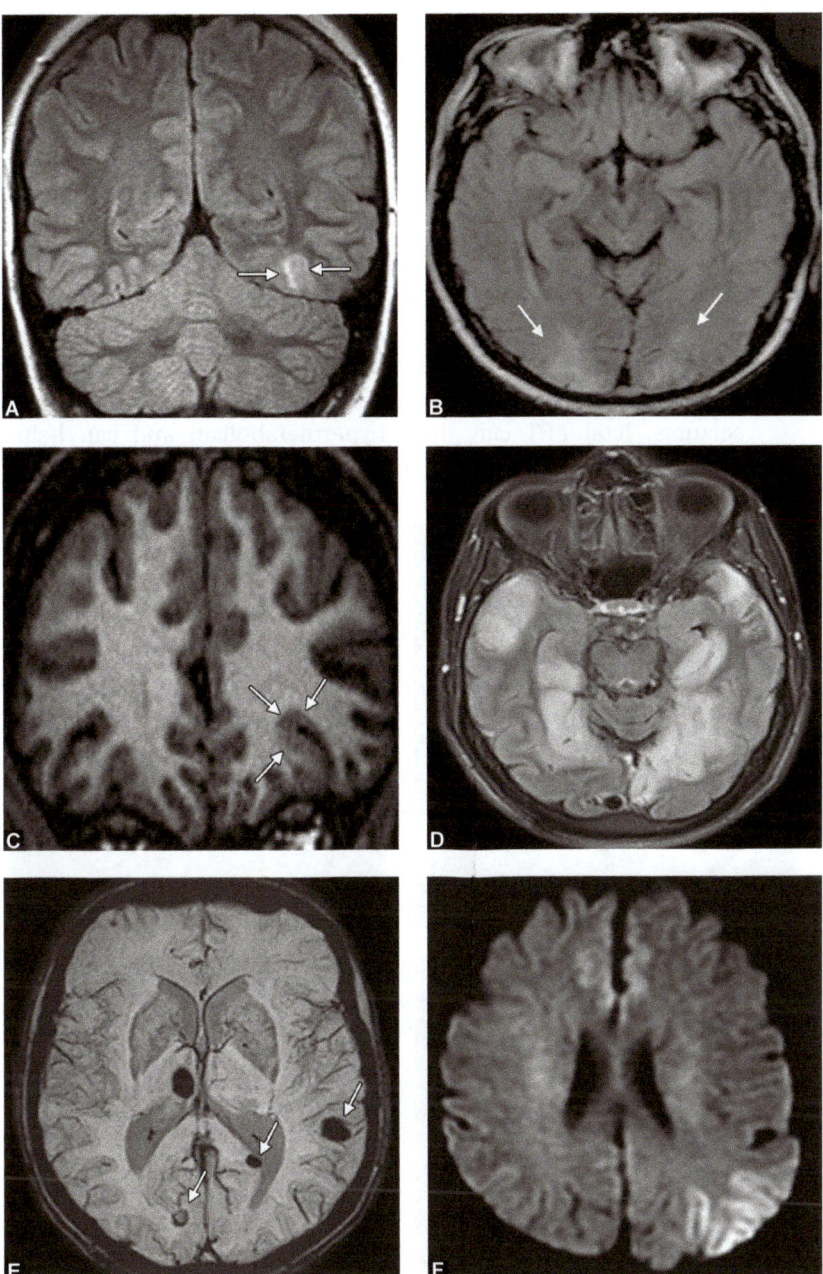

FIG. 6: **A,** coronal fluid-attenuated inversion recovery (FLAIR) showing focal cortical dysplasia; **B,** axial FLAIR showing bilateral occipital gliosis; **C,** coronal T1 images showing sulcal depth cortical dysplasia; **D,** coronal FLAIR showing temporal lobe changes in herpes simplex virus encephalitis; **E,** susceptibility weighted imaging showing calcific lesions; **F,** diffusion MRI showing acute left parietal infarct and seizures

- T1-weighted, T2-weighted, fluid attenuation inversion recovery sequences, three-dimensional coronal and axial sequences, susceptibility weighted images, and T2 relaxometry are usual recommended sequences
- Functional MRI:
  - For localizing motor and sensory cortex and lateralizing language functions (Fig. 7)
- Positron emission tomography (PET) scans:
  - Positron emission tomography scan may be used to locate the part of the brain causing seizures
  - Positron emission tomography scan is usually done in the interictal state and shows hypometabolism in the areas of the brain producing seizures. Ictal PET can show hypermetabolism and can help in localization of seizure focus (Fig. 8).

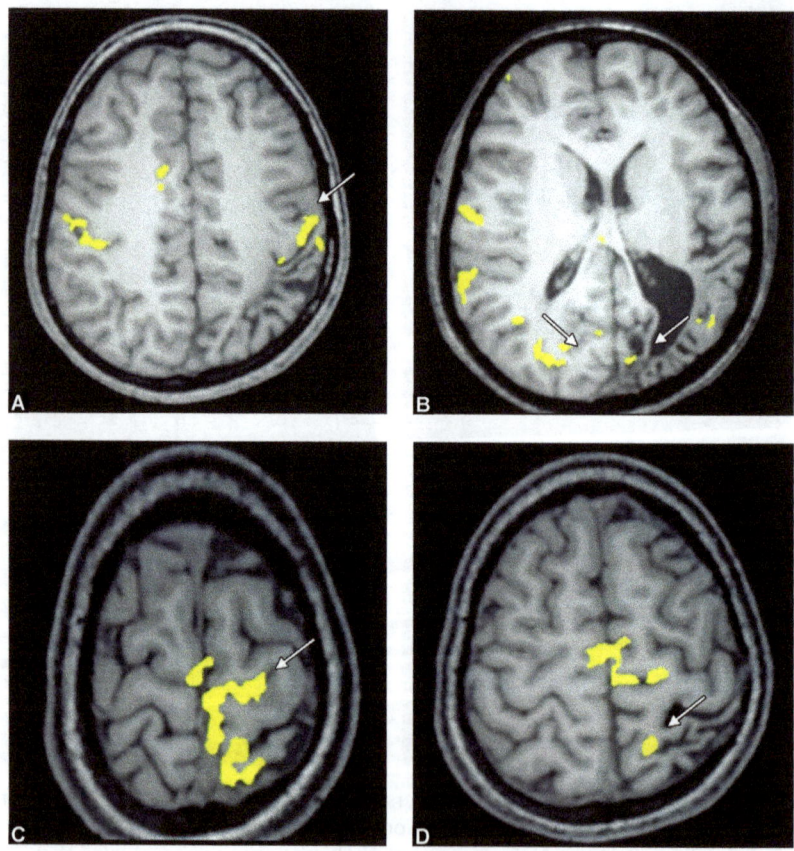

FIG. 7: Functional magnetic resonance imaging images showing blood oxygen level dependent response (yellow maps) **A,** during language **B,** visual cues; **C,** right toe tapping; **D,** right hand motor in a patient with left parieto-occipital gliosis

Epilepsy Diagnosis

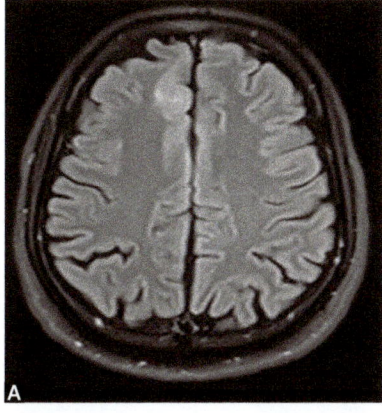
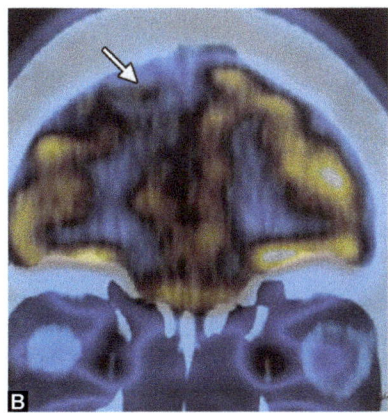
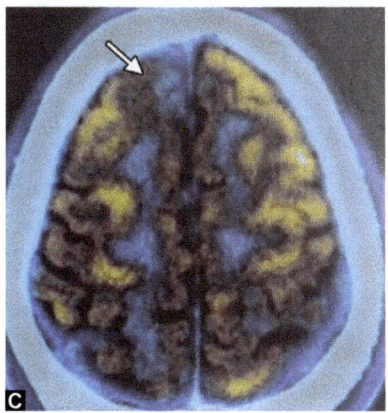

FIG. 8: **A,** Axial magnetic resonance imaging (MRI) showing right mesial frontal cortical dysplasia in patient with medically refractory frontal lobe epilepsy. **B** and **C,** axial and coronal interictal Positron emission tomography–computed tomography brain images showing hypometabolism in right mesial frontal region corresponding to right frontal dysplaasia on MRI

- Single-photon emission computed tomography (SPECT):
  - Functional nuclear imaging technique performed to evaluate regional cerebral perfusion, which is linked to neuronal activity. Pre- and postseizure SPECT scan helps in detection and resection of seizure focus in drug-resistant epilepsy (Fig. 9)
- Magnetoencephalography (MEG):
  - In the evaluation of epilepsy, MEG is used to localize the source of epileptiform brain activity, which most likely is the source of seizures
- Wada test (Amytal study):
  - Also known as the intracarotid sodium amobarbital procedure (ISAP) where sodium amytal or propofol is injected in to the right or left internal carotid artery by placing a catheter and each hemisphere is put to sleep and the contralateral hemisphere, if tested, for memory and language by a neuropsychologist
  - For localization of memory and to lateralizes the language function.

Epilepsy

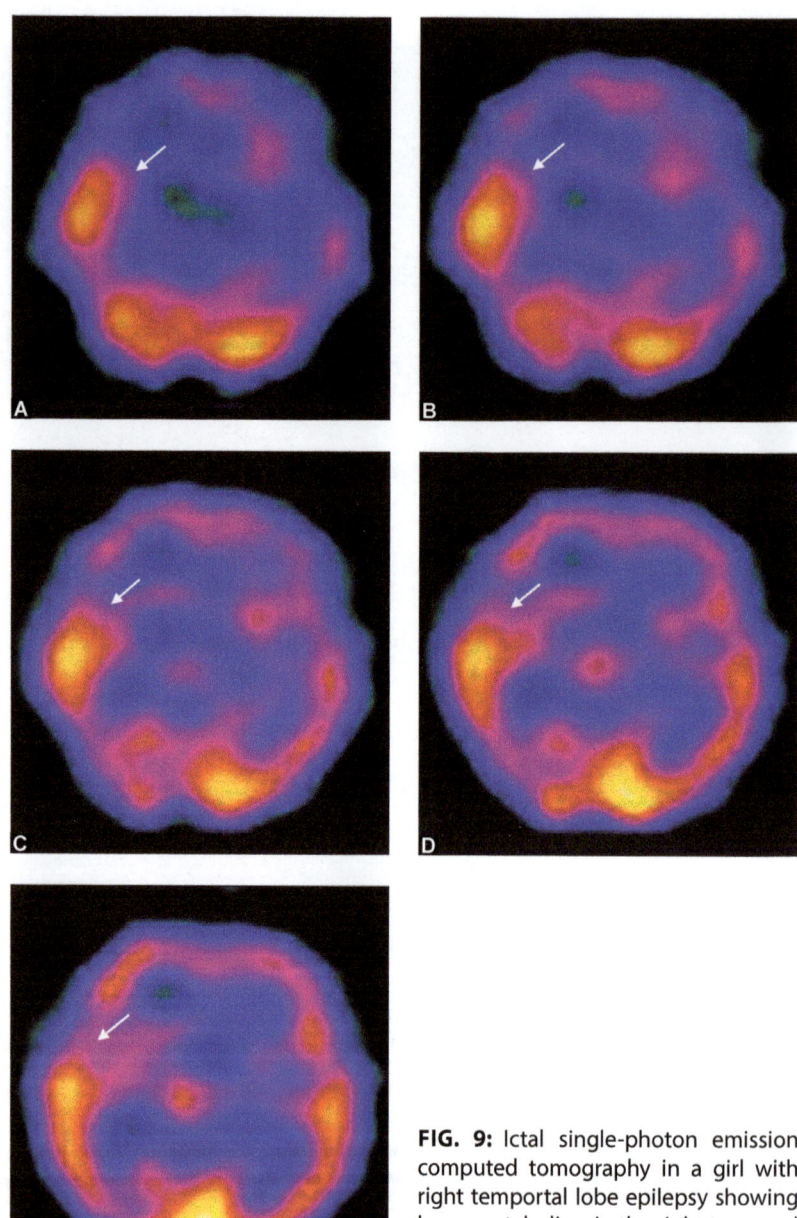

FIG. 9: Ictal single-photon emission computed tomography in a girl with right temporal lobe epilepsy showing hypermetabolism in the right temporal lobe confirming the site of seizure focus

Other Laboratory Tests
- Blood tests:
    - Mainly used in acute exacerbations and evaluation of first seizure:
        – Blood chemistry—sodium and glucose

- Cell counts for infections
- Serum prolactin levels—limited value in differentiating epileptic and nonepileptic seizures
- 25-hydroxy vitamin D levels for bone health status
- Serum levels of anticonvulsants:
  - Carbamazepine, valproic acid, lamotrigine, phenytoin, and phenobarbitone
- To monitor adverse consequences of anticonvulsants:
  - Valproic acid—liver function tests and serum ammonia
  - Phenytoin—bone marrow suppression and osteopenia
- Metabolic workup and genomic testing in suspected metabolic, genetic, and neurodegenerative conditions in children with epilepsy:
  - SCN1A gene is diagnostic of Dravet syndrome
- Cerebrospinal fluid analysis:
  - Suspected neuroinfections
  - Antimeasles antibodies in suspected subacute sclerosing panencephalitis.
- Skin and muscle biopsy:
  - Progressive myoclonic epilepsy
  - Mitochondrial disorders
  - Storage disorders.

CONCLUSION

Diagnosis of epilepsy is clinical and is often based on a detailed description of events experienced by the patient before, during, and after a seizure and more importantly on an eye witness account. In view of the social, psychological, and economic implications and side effects of antiseizure medications, diagnostic errors need to be avoided and minimized. Never make the diagnosis of epilepsy based on suspicion without definite clinical evidence. If there is any doubt, the clinician should wait for further events to clarify the paroxysmal events and to confirm the diagnosis. Electroencephalography and video-EEG help in the classification of seizure type and epilepsy syndrome. If clinical doubt persists, the patient should be referred to an epilepsy center with specialized expertise in diagnosis. Advanced CT and MRI techniques are justified only if new information could lead to change in the course of management like epilepsy surgery and improve the QOLIE patients.

REFERENCES

1. Nowack WJ. Epilepsy: A costly misdiagnosis. Clin Electroencephalogr. 1997;28:225-8.
2. Chowdhury FA, Nashef L, Elwes RD. Misdiagnosis in epilepsy: a review and recognition of diagnostic uncertainty. Eur J Neurol. 2008;15:1034-42.
3. Smith D, Defalla BA, Chadwick DW. The misdiagnosis of epilepsy and the management of refractory epilepsy in a specialist clinic. QJM. 1999;92:15-23.

4. Royal College of Physicians of Edinburgh. Consensus conference on better care for children and adults with epilepsy. Final consensus statement. Edinburgh: The College; 2002.
5. Fisher RS, Acevedo C, Arzimanoglou A, Bogacz A, Cross JH, Elger CE, et al. A practical clinical definition of epilepsy. Epilepsia. 2014;55:475-82.
6. Berg AT, Berkovic SF, Brodie MJ, Buchhalter J, Cross JH, van Emde Boas W, et al. Revised terminology and concepts for organization of seizures and epilepsies: report of the ILAE Commission on Classification and Terminology, 2005-2009. Epilepsia. 2010;51:676-85.
7. Parnell K, Cascino GD, So EL, Cicora K. Long-term EEG monitoring in patients with spells: clinical characteristics and predictive factors. Neurology. 1999;52:A371-2.
8. Benbadis SR, O'Neill E, Tatum WO, Heriaud L. Outcome of prolonged video-EEG monitoring at a typical referral epilepsy center. Epilepsia. 2004;45:1150-3.
9. Stephenson JB. Fits and faints. London: MacKeith Press; 1990.
10. King MA, Newton MR, Jackson GD, Fitt GJ, Mitchell LA, Silvapulle MJ, et al. Epileptology of the first-seizure presentation: a clinical, electroencephalographic, and magnetic resonance imaging study of 300 consecutive patients. Lancet. 1998;352:1007-11.
11. Devinsky O, Sanchez-Villasenor F, Vazquez B, Kothari M, Alper K, Luciano D. Clinical profile of patients with epileptic and nonepileptic seizures. Neurology. 1996;46:1530-3.
12. Doose H, Neubauer BA. Preponderance of female sex in the transmission of seizure liability in idiopathic generalized epilepsy. Epilepsy Res. 2001;43:103-14.
13. Doppelbauer A, Zeitlhofer J, Zifko U, Baumgartner C, Mayr N, Deecke L. Occurrence of epileptiform activity in the routine EEG of epileptic patients. Acta Neurol Scand. 1993;87:345-52.
14. Van Donselaar CA, Schimsheimer RJ, Geerts AT, et al. Value of the electro-encephalogram in adult patients with untreated idiopathic first seizures. Arch Neurol. 1992;49:231-7.
15. Commission on Neuroimaging of the International League Against Epilepsy. Recommendations for neuroimaging of patients with epilepsy. Epilepsia. 1997;38:1255-6.

CHAPTER 5

Approach to the First Episode of Seizure

Rajesh Shankar Iyer

INTRODUCTION

We discuss the approach to evaluation and management of adults with first unprovoked seizure (FUS). We exclude people with epilepsy and restrict ourselves to those with apparent unprovoked first seizure. We conclude by summarizing the various recommendations in the evaluation and management of FUS based on the current evidence.

EVALUATION OF FIRST UNPROVOKED SEIZURE

Role of Electroencephalography

Electroencephalography (EEG) is helpful in the evaluation of an adult with FUS. This is because around 29% of EEGs exhibit significant abnormalities. Seizure recurrence is predicted by these abnormalities.[1] If EEG is done within the first 12 hours of seizure onset, there is a better yield of epileptiform discharges.[2]

Role of Brain Imaging

A computed tomography (CT) or magnetic resonance imaging (MRI) is useful in the evaluation of FUS with a yield of about 10%. It may lead to the diagnosis of disorders like tumor, stroke, and cysticercosis. The detection of these abnormalities has some value in determining the risk for seizure recurrence. Magnetic resonance imaging is more sensitive and likely to show more abnormalities than CT.[3]

Role of Laboratory Investigations

Laboratory investigations like blood counts, sugar, and electrolytes may be ordered based on clinical situations.[4] There is no evidence supporting or negating their routine use.

Lumbar Puncture and Toxicology Screening

Cerebrospinal fluid studies and toxicology studies have been found useful only if clinically indicated and not on a routine basis.

MANAGEMENT

Risk of Seizure Recurrence after First Unprovoked Seizure

Around 21-45% are at risk of a seizure recurrence within the first two years and especially in the first year.[5-8] The risk is lower for patients treated with anti-epileptic drugs (AEDs). The risk of seizure recurrence increases in the following clinical circumstances:
- Electroencephalography with epileptiform abnormalities
- Abnormality in brain imaging
- A prior brain lesion or insult
- Nocturnal seizure.

Immediate Anti-epileptic Drugs Treatment and Short-term Prognosis for Seizure Recurrence

Immediate AED treatment reduces risk of seizure recurrence within the next 2 years by about 35%.[9-11] This, however, may not improve the quality of life.[12] There is also no evidence that use of AEDs reduce mortality.

Immediate Anti-epileptic Drug Treatment and Long-term Prognosis for Seizure Remission

Immediate AED treatment when compared to delayed treatment-pending seizure recurrence is unlikely to affect the chance of attaining sustained seizure remission over 3 years.[13]

Possibility of Adverse Effects of Anti-epileptic Drugs

Mild and reversible adverse effects can occur in 7-31% of patients initiated on AEDs.[14]

RECOMMENDATIONS

The following recommendations are made for evaluation of adults presenting with FUS by the Quality Standards Subcommittee of the American Academy of Neurology (AAN) and the American Epilepsy Society (AES).[15]
- The EEG should be considered as part of the neurodiagnostic evaluation of the adult with FUS because it has a substantial yield and has value in determining the risk of seizure recurrence

- Brain imaging using CT or MRI should be considered
- Blood glucose, blood counts, and electrolyte panels (particularly sodium) may be helpful in specific clinical circumstances, but there are insufficient data to support or refute routine recommendation of any of these laboratory tests
- Lumbar puncture may be helpful in specific clinical circumstances, such as patients who are febrile, but there are insufficient data to support or refute recommending routine lumbar puncture
- Toxicology screening may be helpful in specific clinical circumstances, but there are insufficient data to support or refute a routine recommendation for toxicology screening.

The following recommendations are made for management of adults presenting with FUS by the Guideline Development Subcommittee of the AAN and the AES:[16]

- Adults presenting with FUS should be informed that the chance for a recurrent seizure is greatest within the first 2 years after a first seizure (21–45%)
- Clinical factors associated with an increased risk of seizure recurrence include a prior brain insult such as a stroke or trauma, an EEG with epileptiform abnormalities, a significant brain-imaging abnormality, or a nocturnal seizure
- Clinicians should advise patients that, although immediate AED therapy, as compared with delay of treatment pending a second seizure, is likely to reduce the risk of a seizure recurrence in the 2 years subsequent to a first seizure, it may not improve quality of life
- Clinicians should advise patients that over the longer term (3 years), immediate AED treatment is unlikely to improve the prognosis for sustained seizure remission
- Patients should be advised that their risk for AED-related adverse events range from 7 to 31% and that these events are predominantly mild and reversible.

CONCLUSION

When an adult presents with the first seizure, judicious use of the investigatory modalities is recommended guided by a proper clinical history. When indicated, appropriate AEDs should be initiated. Proper counseling as to the nature of the illness, role of AEDs and their side effects, and long-term prognosis goes a long way in the successful management of an adult with FUS.

REFERENCES

1. Berg AT, Shinnar S. The risk of seizure recurrence following a first unprovoked seizure: a quantitative review. Neurology. 1991;41:965-72.
2. Sofat P, Teter B, Kavak KS, Gupta R, Li P. Time interval providing highest yield for initial EEG in patients with new onset seizures. Epilepsy Res. 2016;127:229-32.
3. Greenberg MK, Barson WG, Starkman S. Practice parameter: Neuroimaging in the emergency patient presenting with a seizure. Neurology. 1996;47:26-32.
4. Edmondstone WM. How do we manage the first seizure in adults? J R Coll Phys Lond. 1995;29:289-94.
5. Hauser WA, Rich SS, Annegers JF, Anderson VE. Seizure recurrence after a 1st unprovoked seizure: an extended follow-up. Neurology. 1990;40:1163-70.
6. Hopkins A, Garman A, Clarke C. The first seizure in adult life: value of clinical features, electroencephalography, and computerised tomographic scanning in prediction of seizure recurrence. Lancet. 1988;1:721-6.
7. Bora I, Seckin B, Zarifoglu M, Turan F, Sadikoglu S, Ogul E. Risk of recurrence after first unprovoked tonic-clonic seizure in adults. J Neurol. 1995;242:157-63.
8. Berg AT. Risk of recurrence after a first unprovoked seizure. Epilepsia. 2008;49:13-8.
9. First Seizure Trial Group (FIRST Group). Randomized clinical trial on the efficacy of antiepileptic drugs in reducing the risk of relapse after a first unprovoked tonic-clonic seizure. Neurology. 1993;43:478-83.
10. Musicco M, Behgi E, Solari A, Viani F; First Seizure Trial Group (FIRST Group). Treatment of first tonic-clonic seizure does not improve the prognosis of epilepsy. Neurology. 1997;49:991-8.
11. Marson A, Jacoby A, Johnson A, Kim L, Gamble C, Chadwick D, et al. Immediate versus deferred antiepileptic drug treatment for early epilepsy and single seizures: a randomized controlled trial. Lancet. 2005;365:2007-13.
12. Jacoby A, Gamble C, Doughty J, Marson A, Chadwick D; Medical Research Council MESS Study Group. Quality of life outcomes of immediate or delayed treatment of early epilepsy and single seizures. Neurology. 2007;68:1188-96.
13. Leone MA, Solari A, Beghi E; FIRST Group. Treatment of the first tonic-clonic seizure does not affect the long-term remission of epilepsy. Neurology. 2006;67:2227-9.
14. Perruca P, Jacoby A, Marson AG, Baker GA, Lane S, Benn EK, et al. Adverse antiepileptic drug effects in new-onset seizures: a case control study. Neurology. 2011;76:273-9.
15. Krumholz A, Wiebe S, Gronseth G, Shinnar S, Levisohn P, Ting T. et al. Practice parameter: evaluating an apparent unprovoked first seizure in adults (an evidence-based review): report of the Quality Standards Subcommittee of the American Academy of Neurology and the American Epilepsy Society. Neurology. 2007;69:1996-2007.
16. Krumholz A, Wiebe S, Gronseth GS, Gloss DS, Sanchez AM, Kabir AA, et al. Evidence-based guideline: management of an unprovoked first seizure in adults: Report of the Guideline Development Subcommittee of the American Academy of Neurology and the American Epilepsy Society. Neurology. 2015;84:1705-13.

CHAPTER 6

Epilepsy Pharmacotherapy: The Anti-epileptic Drugs

Mugundhan Krishnan

INTRODUCTION

Epilepsy and seizures cause morbidity and sometimes mortality unless managed appropriately. Most cases of epilepsy can be controlled using drugs. The knowledge of the anti-epiletpic drugs (AEDs) used, their mechanism of action and adverse effects helps in identifying appropriate treatment modality and decision of choice of AED. Further, the usage of AED in special situations where the co-morbid conditions are a concern is a challenge and this is also discussed.

MANAGEMENT OF EPILEPSY

Anti-epileptic drugs are the main form of treatment for people with epilepsy; up to 70% people with epilepsy could have their seizures controlled with AEDs. There are many AEDs used to treat seizures, and different AEDs work for different seizures. Here we explain what the different AEDs are what type of seizures or epilepsy, they are used for as well as some essential information about average doses and common side effects.

CLASSIFICATION OF ANTI-EPILEPTIC DRUGS

Cyclic Ureides

- Phenytoin and fosphenytoin
- Primidone
- Phenobarbital
- Ethosuximide.

Tricyclics

- Carbamazepine
- Oxcarbazepine
- Eslicarbazepine.

Benzodiazepines
- Diazepam
- Clonazepam
- Lorazepam
- Clobazam.

Gamma-Aminobutyric Acid Derivatives
- Gabapentin
- Pregabalin
- Vigabatrin.

Other
- Valproate
- Lamotrigine
- Levetiracetam
- Retigabine
- Rufinamide
- Tiagabine
- Topiramate
- Zonisamide
- Lacosamide
- Perampanel.

Antiseizure drugs act by one of the three mechanisms:
1. Enhancement of inhibitory transmission [γ-aminobutyric acid (GABA)-ergic]
2. Diminution of excitatory transmission (usually glutaminergic)
3. Modification of ionic conductances.

Molecular Targets at the Excitatory Synapse

Presynaptic Targets

Voltage-gated Sodium Channels
- Phenytoin
- Carbamazepine
- Lamotrigine
- Lacosamide.

Voltage-gated Calcium Channels
- Ethosuximide
- Lamotrigine
- Gabapentin

Epilepsy Pharmacotherapy: The Anti-epileptic Drugs

- Pregabalin
- K⁺ channels (retigabine)
- Synaptic vesicle proteins (SV2A)—levetiracetam
- Collapsin response mediator protein-2 (CRMP2).

Postsynaptic Targets

Alpha-amino-3-hydroxy-5-methyl-4-isoxazole propionic acid (AMPA) receptors

- Phenobarbital
- Topiramate
- Lamotrigine
- Peramapanel.

N-methyl-D-aspartate (NMDA) receptors
Felbamate.

Molecular Targets at the Inhibitory Synapse

- GABA transporters (GAT1)—tiagabine
- GABA transaminase—vigabatrin
- GABA-A receptors—benzodiazepines
- GABA-B receptors.

Phenytoin

Mechanism of Action

Phenytoin acts by preferential binding to sodium channel and prolongation of its inactivated state. It also decreases the synaptic release of glutamate and enhance the releases of GABA

Uses

- Partial seizures
- Generalized tonic-clonic seizures (GTCS).

Pharmacokinetics

- *Absorption*: From gastrointestinal tract is nearly complete in most patients
- Highly bound to plasma proteins[1]
- Elimination is dose dependent
- Therapeutic plasma level: 10–20 μg/mL.

Drug Interactions

Due to:
- High-protein binding
- Induce microsomal enzymes.

Adverse Effects

Dose related:
- Nystagmus, diplopia, ataxia, gum hyperplasia and hirsutism
- Peripheral neuropathy, osteomalacia and megaloblastic anemia.

Phenobarbital

Mechanism of Action

Enhances phasic GABA-A receptor responses and also reduces excitatory synaptic responses.[2]

Uses

- Partial seizures
- Generalized tonic-clonic seizures
- Myoclonic seizures
- Generalized seizures
- Neonatal seizures
- Status epilepticus.

Pharmacokinetics

Nearly complete absorption, not significantly bound to plasma proteins. Peak concentrations in 0.5-4 hours and no active metabolites. $T_{1/2}$ varies from 75-125 hour. Therapeutic plasma level: 10-40 μg/mL.

Adverse Effects

Sedation, cognitive issues, hyperactivity and ataxia.

Valproate

Mechanism of Action

Valproate blocks sustained high-frequency repetitive firing of neurons as a consequence of its effect on sodium currents. Blockade of NMDA receptor-mediated excitation has also been seen. Facilitation of glutamic acid decarboxylase (GAD—GABA synthesis enzyme), inhibitory effect on GAT1 and inhibition of GABA transaminase result in enhanced level of GABA in brain.

Indications

Very effective in the management of absence seizures, certain myoclonic seizures, GTCS and atonic attacks. It is also being used in the management of bipolar disorder and prophylaxis of migraine.[3]

Dosage

30-60 mg/kg/day.

Epilepsy Pharmacotherapy: The Anti-epileptic Drugs

Adverse Effects
- Dose related—nausea, vomiting, gastrointestinal (GI) complaints, weight gain and hair loss
- Idiosyncratic—hepatotoxicity (risk being greater for infants <2 years), thrombocytopenia and teratogenicity.

Benzodiazepines
Diazepam
Mechanism of action: Potentiates GABA-A responses

Uses
- Status epilepticus
- Seizure clusters.

Pharmacokinetics
Well-absorbed oral, rectal administration gives peak concentration in 1 hour with 90% bioavailability, can be given intravenous for status epilepticus, highly protein bound, extensively metabolized to several active metabolites[4] and has a half-life of 2 days.

Route
Parenteral and rectal.

Adverse Effects
Sedation.

Carbamazepine
Mechanism of Action
- Blocks Na⁺ channels and inhibits high-frequency firing of neurons. Potentiation of voltage-gated K⁺ channels
- Therapeutic level: 4–8 μg/mL.

Uses
- GTCS
- Partial seizures
- Drug interactions mainly due to enzyme-inducing properties.

Adverse Effects
- *Dose related*—diplopia, ataxia, GI symptoms and hyponatremia
- *Idiosyncratic reactions*—agranulocytosis, aplastic anemia, erythematous skin rash and hepatic dysfunction.

Oxcarbazepine: Less potent, but less interactions.

Eslicarbazepine: Once daily dosing regimen.

Felbamate

Mechanism of Action
- NMDA receptor blocker (NR1-2B subtype)
- Potentiation of GABA-A receptor responses.

Uses
- Partial seizures
- Lennox-Gastaut syndrome.[5]

Adverse Effects
- Aplastic anemia
- Severe hepatitis.

Dosage
- 2–4 g/day
- Effective plasma level: 30–100 µg/mL.

Gamma-amino Butyric Acid Analogs—Gabapentin and Pregabalin

Mechanism of Action
Modify the release of GABA, by binding to the α-2 δ-subunit of voltage-gated N-type calcium channels, thereby decreasing calcium entry in the presynaptic channels. The anti-epileptic effect is brought about by decrease in the synaptic release of glutamate.

Uses
It is used as an adjunct against partial as well as GTCS. It is also found to be useful in neuropathic pain as in postherpetic neuralgia and diabetic peripheral neuropathy. Pregabalin is the first drug to be approved for fibromyalgia in the USA. Its usefulness in generalized anxiety disorder is also being explored.

Adverse Effects
Somnolence, dizziness, ataxia, tremors and headache.

Lacosamide

An amino acid related compound useful in the treatment of partial seizures.

Mechanism of Action
It enhances the slow inactivation of voltage-gated sodium channels. Previously binding to CRMP2 receptor and blocking the effect of growth factors like brain-derived neurotrophic factor and NT3 were thought to occur. However, recent studies are against this theory.[6]

Epilepsy Pharmacotherapy: The Anti-epileptic Drugs

Uses
It has been found useful as an adjunctive therapy in the management of partial onset seizures.

Dosage
- 200 mg/day, typically twice daily dosing
- *Formulations*: Oral and intravenous form are available.

Lamotrigine

Mechanism of Action
It suppresses rapid firing of neurons, much like the action of lamotrigine, producing blockade of voltage-gated Na^+ channels. In addition, inhibits voltage-gated calcium channels, both N- and P/Q-type, making it useful in absence seizures and primary generalized seizures in childhood. Decrease in the synaptic release of glutamate has also been found to be another mechanism.

Uses
- As monotherapy in partial seizures
- For control of seizures in Lennox-Gastaut syndrome
- Activity against absence and myoclonic seizures in children has also been found
- Bipolar disorder.

Adverse Effects
- Hypersensitivity rash, which may be more in pediatric population. The risk of developing rash may be diminished by slow introduction of the drug.
- Dizziness, headache, somnolence, diplopia and nausea are other adverse effects.

Dosage
- 100–300 mg/day
- Therapeutic blood level µg/mL.

Levetiracetam

Piracetam analog that is used as an anti-epileptic.

Mechanism of Action
It binds selectively to the synaptic vesicular protein SV2A, thereby releasing the release of glutamate and GABA. Inhibition of N-type calcium channels, decreasing the release of calcium from intracellular stores is an additional mode of action.

Uses

It is used for the adjunctive treatment of partial seizures and for myoclonic seizures in Juvenile myoclonic epilepsy.

Dosage

Begin with 500 or 1,000 mg/day (twice daily dosing) up to a maximum of 3,000 mg/day.

Adverse Effects

Somnolence, asthenia, ataxia, mood and behavioral changes, and rarely, psychotic reactions.[7]

Formulations

Oral and intravenous.

Pharmacokinetics

Oral absorption of the drug is complete and rapid, unaffected by food. It follows a linear kinetics. Plasma half-life is 6–8 hours. The drug has minimal interactions. It is excreted unchanged in the urine.

Tiagabine

Mechanism of Action

It is an inhibitor of GABA uptake in both neurons and glia, by preferential inhibition of the transporter GAT1. This increases the extracellular concentration of GABA, mainly in the forebrain and hippocampus. Increased levels of GABA result in potentiation of tonic inhibition.

Uses

Indicated for the adjunctive treatment of partial seizures.

Dosage

16–56 mg/day.

Adverse Effects

- Dose related—tremor, dizziness, difficulty in concentration, depression and rarely psychosis
- Idiosyncratic—rash.

Topiramate

Mechanism of Action

Blockage of voltage-gated sodium channels and L-type calcium channels thereby blocking the repetitive firing of neurons. Potentiation of the

Epilepsy Pharmacotherapy: The Anti-epileptic Drugs

inhibitory effect of GABA has also been observed, at a site different from that of benzodiazepines or barbiturates. It also depresses the excitatory action of kainate on glutamate receptors.[8] The multiple effects of topiramate are postulated to have a result through a primary action on kinase, altering the phosphorylation of voltage-gated and ligand-gated ion channels.

Uses
It may be used as monotherapy against partial and GTCS. It is also approved for Lennox-Gastaut syndrome, infantile spasms and even absent seizures. It can also be used for treatment of migraine.

Dosage
200–600 mg/day.

Adverse Effects
- Mostly dose related: Somnolence, dizziness, cognitive slowing, paresthesia and confusion
- Acute myopia and glaucoma may warrant drug withdrawal. Urolithiasis has also been reported. Teratogenicity is being explored.

Vigabatrin

Mechanism of Action
Irreversible inhibitor of GABA transaminase producing a sustained increase in the extracellular concentration of GABA in the brain and secondary decrease in the brain glutamine synthetase activity.

Uses
Useful in the treatment of partial seizures and infantile spasms.

Dosage
- *Infants*—50–150 mg/day
- *Adults*—Started with 500 mg twice daily to a maximum of 2–3 g.

Adverse Effects
Drowsiness, dizziness, weight gain, agitation, confusion and psychosis. Pre-existing mental illness is a relative contraindication. Long-term therapy with vigabatrin has been associated with development of peripheral visual field defect in 30–50% of patients (usually not reversible).[9]

Zonisamide

It is a sulfonamide derivative.

Mechanism of Action
Acts on the sodium channel and T-type voltage-gated channels.

Uses

Partial seizures, GTCS, infantile spasms and myoclonias.[1]

Dosage
- *Children*—4-12 mg/day
- *Adult*—100-600 mg/day.

Adverse Effects

Drowsiness, cognitive impairment and skin rashes.

Ethosuximide

Mechanism of Action

Reducing the low threshold (T-type) calcium current mainly in the thalamic neurons. The T-type calcium currents are thought to be responsible for generating the rhythmic cortical discharge of an absence attack, accounting for the specific therapeutic action of ethosuximide.

Uses

It is used in absence seizures.

Dosage

750–1,500 mg/day.

Adverse Effects

Gastric distress, transient lethargy, hiccups and euphoria.

Acetazolamide

Mechanism of Action

Inhibition of carbonic anhydrase causing mild acidosis in the brain.[10]

Uses

It has been used for all type of seizures.

Perampanel

Mechanism of Action

It is an AMPA antagonist, which binds to an allosteric site on the glutamate-gated Na⁺/K⁺ AMPA channel, and hence preventing repetitive discharge—noncompetitive blockade.

Uses

Approved for the adjunctive treatment of partial seizures with or without secondary generalization in patients more than 12 years. Though FDA approved its use in 2011, this drug is currently not available in India.

Dosage

4–12 mg/day (once daily dosing).

Adverse Effects

Serious behavioral adverse reactions (aggression, hostility, etc.), dizziness, somnolence, headache and benign transient rash.

Retigabine (Ezogabine)

Relatively newer drug which was approved by FDA in 2012 however, the drug is not available for clinical use in India.

Mechanism of Action

Unique mechanism—potassium-channel facilitator.

Uses

Adjunctive treatment for partial onset seizures in adults.

Dosage

600–1,200 mg/day (thrice daily administration).

Adverse Effects

Most are dose related, and include dizziness, somnolence, blurred vision, confusion and dysarthria. Bladder dysfunction was noted in many trials. Bluish pigmentation of the skin and lips, and retinal pigment abnormalities are other disturbing adverse effects, which may be permanent. The development of these adverse effects may be reasons to discontinue the drug.

Rufinamide

Mechanism of Action

It decreases high-frequency firing of neurons, by prolonging the inactive state of Na^+ channels.

Uses

It has been approved for the adjunctive treatment of seizures associated with Lennox-Gastaut syndrome in patients older than 4 years of age. It is effective in all types of seizures in this syndrome.[11] The drug has also been marketed in India.

Dosage

Treatment is initiated with 10 mg/kg/day up to a maximum of 45 mg/kg/day. Maximum dose is 3,200 mg/day. Twice daily administration of the drug is thought to be the best.

Adverse Effects

Somnolence, vomiting, pyrexia and diarrhea.

Stiripentol

Mechanism of Action

It is not clearly understood; mainly by augmenting GABAergic transmission in the brain, by prolonging the opening of calcium channels in GABA-A receptors. It can increase the effect of other AEDs by slowing their interaction by cytochrome P450.

Uses

It is used with clobazam and valproate in the adjunctive therapy of refractory GTCS in patients with severe myoclonic epilepsy of infancy (SMEI-Dravet's syndrome), when the convulsions cannot be controlled with clobazam and valproate. Though used in European countries, it is not approved by FDA.

Dosage

Reduction of the concomitant medication is the first step while initiating treatment. Initial dose of the drug is 10 mg/kg/day, which is gradually increased to higher doses.

MANAGEMENT OF EPILEPSY IN PERSONS WITH COMORBID CONDITIONS

The prevalence of comorbid conditions such as diabetes, heart diseases, systemic hypertension, bronchial asthma, cancers, thyroid disorders, etc. was found to be higher in patients with epilepsy.[12] Besides, mental health disorders are also common in epileptic patients.[13] These comorbid conditions can be a cause of the epilepsy itself (e.g., stroke) or have no apparent relation to epilepsy. Despite these facts, no universal guidelines are available for treatment of epilepsy in those patients with comorbidities.

Cardiovascular Diseases

In case of administration of phenytoin in for acute seizure patients with cardiovascular disease, caution should be exercised so that the dose does not to exceed 10 mg/min administration since rapid administration can lead to arrhythmias. Preferable, cardiac monitoring and blood pressure monitoring should be done.[14] Administration of intravenous fosphenytoin and phenytoin should be avoided in patients with severe cardiac disease or high-degree heart blocks. Diazepam with proper respiratory monitoring and sodium valproate are better alternatives in these situations. In chronic management, carbamazepine and related drugs and phenytoin should be used carefully and should be avoided in patients with heart blocks. Pregabalin worsens left ventricular function and should be used carefully. The most recommended AEDs are lamotrigine, topiramate, valproic acid (VPA), and zonisamide with gabapentin, which can be used as an adjunct.

Lung Diseases

Administration of barbiturates, benzodiazepines and phenytoin parenterally can cause respiratory depression. When they are used, careful monitoring of respiratory and heart rate along with emergency cardiorespiratory resuscitation equipment should be available. Enzyme inducers in AEDs can reduce the level of theophylline, which in-turn can reduce the levels of carbamazepine and phenytoin.

Liver Diseases

Hypoalbuminemia and impaired drug metabolism of certain drugs in liver necessitates drug-dose adjustment in liver disorders. If liver disease is mild, there need not be any dose adjustment. Usage of phenobarbitone and benzodiazepines may trigger hepatic encephalopathy, and hence should only be used very cautiously and in lower doses when indicated absolutely.[15]

Phenytoin due to its high-protein binding needs to be used cautiously because the free fraction increases in hypoalbuminemia leading to toxicity. Drugs for chronic treatment are levetiracetam, oxcarbazepine, pregabalin and topiramate due to their limited liver metabolism and dose adjustment is needed even in these drugs in case of severe liver disease. Lamotrigine and VPA are not recommended.

Kidney Disease

In renal impairment, levetiracetam is contraindicated since it is eliminated through kidneys. Chronic use of gabapentin, levetiracetam, phenobarbitone, topiramate, oxcarbazepine and zonisamide needs to be cautious since these are eliminated through kidneys-requiring dose adjustment. Those on hemodialysis and in those with renal impairment, the recommended drugs are those that are metabolized in liver, e.g., benzodiazepines, carbamazepine, phenytoin, VPA, trigabine and ethosuximide.[16]

Porphyria

Drugs of choice are gabapentin, levetiracetam and pregabalin and those contraindicated are enzyme inducers including carbamazepine, phenytoin, phenobarbitone, VPA, etc.

Thyroid Disorders

Enzyme-inducing AEDs (carbamazepine, phenobarbitone, phenytoin and primidone) can influence the hormone metabolism and cause decrease in total and free-thyroxin levels, which may be significant in hypothyroid individuals.

Transplant Recipients

The following issues need to be considered in choosing AED in patients who are organ recipients:
- Hepatic or renal impairment in patients who received liver or kidney transplant
- Drug interaction with immunosuppressants, which may be adverse by reducing the levels of cyclosporine, sirolimus and steroids, necessitating the increase in dose of these drugs. Azathioprine, mycophenolate and OKT3 are not significantly affected by AED
- Valproic acid should be avoided in liver transplant recipients; carbamazepine, phenobarbital and primidone should be avoided in bone marrow transplant cases.[17]

With above considerations, drugs which can be used include gabapentin, levetiracetam, pregabalin and topiramate can be used.

Metabolic Disorders

- Enzyme inducers accelerate vitamin D catabolism and increase bone turnover and VPA interferes with osteoblasts
- Some AEDs are associated with weight gain such as carbamazepine, gabapentin, and some drugs such as topiramate and zonisamide can cause weight loss. Majority are weight neutral.

Infections

Praziquantel and albendazole levels are decreased by enzyme inducers by about 50%. Rifampicin reduces the plasma levels of AEDs such as carbamazepine, tage lamotrigine, phenobarbitone, VPA and phenytoin. VPA may sometimes increase the replication of latent HIV in vitro, but there is no evidence against its use.[18]

Mental Disability and Psychiatric Illness

Studies reveal that there is a higher incidence of seizures in patients with mental disorders and drugs with potential to cause cognitive impairment and sedation are to be avoided for long-term use like gabapentin, levetiracetam, lamotrigine, oxcarbazepine and VPA. In psychiatric illness, the potential for the used drug to influence the underlying psychiatric illness need to be considered. Further, the plasma levels may be increased (VPA can cause nortriptyline level to increase by 60%) leading to toxicity or may lead to reduction (tricyclics, neruoleptics and serotonin reuptake inhibitors may decrease with enzyme-inducing AED) leading to suboptimal therapeutic response.

Stroke

Conventional AEDs such as benzodiazepines, carbamazepine, phenytoin or phenobarbitone are not preferred due to the fact that they may lead to delayed functional recovery.[19] Gabapentin and levetiracetam are preferred in patients with stroke.

Brain Tumors

In glioblastoma multiforme, enzyme-inducing AEDs reduce survival. VPA is conventional drug of choice. Levetiracetam has shown good results and tolerated better. Lamotrigine is a good drug for focal seizures. Pregabalin and zonisamide are alternatives for treatment of epilepsy in brain tumor patients.[20]

CONCLUSION

The fact that AEDs are the cornerstone in management of epilepsy makes it imperative that the proper selection of drugs based on the type of seizure and possible side-effects which may affect the quality of life are to taken into consideration. Appropriate selection of drugs based on the patient profile taking into consideration the co-morbidities helps in ensuring adequate control of the symptoms and improve quality of life without compromising on safety of question of adherence.

REFERENCES

1. French JA, Wang S, Warnock B, Temkin N. Historical control monotherapy design in the treatment of epilepsy. Epilepsia. 2010:51:1936-43.
2. Avorn J. Drug warnings that can cause fits-communicating risks in a data poor environment. N Engl J Med. 2008;359:991-4.
3. Potter RJ, Baulac M, Nohria V. Clinical development of drugs for epilepsy: a review of approaches in the United States and Europe. Epilepsy Res. 2010;89:163-75.
4. French JA, White HS, Klitgaard H, Holmes GL, Privitera MD, Cole AJ, et al. Development of new treatment approaches for epilepsy: unmet needs and opportunities. Epilepsia. 2013;54:3-12.
5. Meldrum BS, Rogawsky MA. Molecular targets for antiepileptic drug development. Neurotherapeutics. 2007;4:18-61.
6. Cross SA, Curran MP. Lacosamide: in partial onset seizures. Drugs. 2009;69:449-59.
7. Lynch BA, Lambeng N, Nocka K, et al. The synaptic vesicle protein SV2A is the binding site for the antiepileptic drug levetiracetam. Proc Natl Acad Sci USA. 2004.

8. Steinhof BJ, Ben-Menachem E, Ryvlin P, Shorvon S, Kramer L, Satlin A, et al. Efficacy and safety of adjunctive perampanel for the treatment of refractory partial seizures: a pooled analysis of three phase III studies. Epilepsia. 2013;54:1481-9.
9. Wilcox KS, Dixon-Salazar T, Sills GJ, Ben-Menachem E, White HS, Porter RJ, et al. Issues related to development of new anti-seizures treatments. Epilepsia. 2013;54:24-34.
10. Glauser TA, Cnaan A, Shinnar S, Hirtz DG, Dlugos D, Masur D, et al. Ethosuximide, valproic acid, and lamotrigine in childhood absence epilepsy. N Engl J Med. 2010;362:790-9.
11. Molgaard-Nielsen D, Hviid A. Newer-generation antiepileptic drugs and the risk of major birth defects. JAMA. 2011;305:1996-2002.
12. Tellez-Zenteno JF, Matijevic S, Wiebe S. Somatic comorbidity of epilepsy in the general population in Canada. Epilepsia. 2005;46:1955-62.
13. Tellez-Zenteno JF, Patten SB, Jetté N, Williams J, Wiebe S. Psychiatric comorbidity in epilepsy: a population-based analysis. Epilepsia. 2007;48:2336-44.
14. Donovan PJ, Cline D. Phenytoin administration by constant intravenous infusion: selective rates of administration. Ann Emerg Med. 1991;20:139-42.
15. Ochs HR, Greenblatt DJ, Eckardt B, Harmatz JS, Shader RI. Repeated diazepam dosing in cirrhotic patients: cumulation and sedation. Clin Pharmacol Ther. 1983;33:471-6.
16. Israni RK, Kasbekar N, Haynes K, Berns JS. Use of antiepileptic drugs in patients with kidney disease. Semin Dialysis. 2006;19:408-16.
17. Focosi D, Kast RE, Benedetti E, Papineschi F, Galimberti S, Petrini M. Phenobarbital-associated bone marrow aplasia: a case report and review of the literature. Acta Haematol. 2008;119:18-21.
18. Sagot-Lerolle N, Lamine A, Chaix ML, Boufassa F, Aboulker JP, Costagliola D, et al. Prolonged valproic acid treatment does not reduce the size of latent HIV reservoir. AIDS. 2008;22:1125-9.
19. Goldstein B. Common drugs may influence motor recovery after stroke. Neurology. 1995;45:865-71.
20. Novy J, Stupp R, Rossetti AO. Pregabalin in patients with primary brain tumors and seizures: a preliminary observation. Clin Neurol Neurosurg. 2009;111:171-3.

7
CHAPTER

Epilepsy and Women

Neeraj N Baheti, Atma Ram Bansal

INTRODUCTION

Approximately half of all persons with epilepsy are women. It is well-known that women with epilepsy have a number of special issues to consider. The changing balance of hormones throughout life complicates the treatment of epilepsy in women. Epilepsy and anti-epileptic drugs (AEDs) substantially affect women's health in the areas of menstruation, sexual function, fertility, contraception, reproduction and bone health.[1] This chapter covers major issues faced by women with epilepsy (WWE) and aims to provides the reader guidelines for clinical care of females with epilepsy.

EPILEPSY AND MENSTRUATION

Catamenial Epilepsy

Catamenial epilepsy is cyclic exacerbation of seizures in relation to menstrual cycle.[2] It is defined as doubling of seizure frequency in relation to a particular phase of the menstrual cycle.[3] The prevalence is around 35% of focal epilepsies. The catamenial seizure worsening is based on three factors:
- The properties of neuroactive steroids, estrogen being neuroexcitatory versus progesterone and its metabolite being neuroinhibitory
- The susceptibility of epileptic substrate to neuroactive steroids
- The variations in the levels of neuroactive steroids during the menstrual cycle (estrogen in the first half vs. progesterone in the second half).

The normal 28 days cycle (with day 14 representing ovulation) is divided into follicular phase (days 1 to 14) and the luteal phase (day –14 to –1). There are three commonly determined patterns of catamenial epilepsy (Table 1). Careful tracking of seizure frequency, menstrual cycles, and, ideally, ovulation is essential to make a diagnosis of catamenial epilepsy.

TABLE 1: Patterns of catamenial epilepsy

Type	Pattern	Cause
C1	Perimenstrual: Days –3 to 3 of the next cycle	Perimenstrual progesterone withdrawal
C2	Periovulatory: Days 10 to –13	Mid-cycle estrogen surge
C3	Luteal phase: days 10 to 3 of the next cycle	High estrogen levels to progesterone ratio due to anovulatory cycle

Treatment of Catamenial Epilepsy

Current approaches to the treatment of catamenial epilepsy are based on small, non-blinded studies and/or on anecdotal reports of success. No There is no US Food and Drug Administration (FDA) approved drug for catamenial epilepsy Several adjunctive medications can be given as intermittent therapy targeting the catamenial patterns are acetazolamide, clobazam and natural progesterone.[4]

Intermittent Therapy for Catamenial Epilepsy

- Acetazolamide
  - 250–1,000 mg in two divided doses
  - Intermittent therapy (± 4 days around periovulatory or perimenstrual period)
- Clobazam
  - 10–20 mg single daily
  - ± 4 days around periovulatory or perimenstrual period
- Natural progesterone (C3 pattern)
  - 100–200 mg TID
  - Day 14–25 of cycle followed by 3-days taper-off.

Polycystic Ovarian Syndrome

Polycystic ovarian syndrome (PCOS) is the most common endocrine disorder in women of reproductive age. The incidence of PCOS is 10-25% in WWE which is significantly higher than in women in general population (~5%).[5] Polycystic ovarian syndrome is diagnosed in presence of two of three following symptoms:
- Oligomenorrhea, anovulation
- Hyperandrogenism
- Polycystic ovaries (>10 ovarian cysts in a single ultrasound plane measuring 2-8 mm in diameter) on ultrasound scan.[6]

Elevated androgen levels, increase in luteinizing hormone (LH) to follicle-stimulating hormone (FSH) ratio, elevated cholesterol, elevated fasting insulin levels, and glucose levels are the biochemical features of PCOS. Long-term consequences of PCOS include infertility, dyslipidemia, glucose intolerance and diabetes, and endometrial cancer. Treatment with valproate significantly increases the incidence of PCOS.[7] Substitution of valproate with other AED usually reverses the effects.[8]

Contraception

Nearly 40% of women with epilepsy have unplanned pregnancies, at times posing a risk to the mother and the fetus.[9] All female patients should have full information regarding effective contraception so as to consider best suitable option for her.

Hormonal oral contraceptive pill (OCP) use is complicated in WWE complicated because of bidirectional pharmacokinetic interactions, pharmacodynamic consequences, and potential effects on seizure control (Table 2).[10] Enzyme inducing AEDs (EIAEDs) reduce serum estrogen concentration by 40–50%. They also increase the serum concentration of the sex hormone binding globulin, thus reducing the level of free progesterone. WWE on enzyme inducing AEDs have increased risk of failure with OCPs or other hormonal forms of birth control (e.g., vaginal ring, patch). Progesterone only OCP are also not reliable. If at all to be used, the hormonal contraceptive pill should contain at least 50 μg estrogen. One should warn patients that mid-cycle bleeding indicates possible OCP failure and alternative contraception should be used for the remainder cycle. At time, ovulation can happen without this warning even.

Barriers or IUDs are better preferred contraceptive methods in WWE.

Levonorgestrel-containing IUD (Mirena) prevents pregnancy by local hormonally-mediated changes in cervical mucus and is not likely to be impacted by enzyme-inducing AEDs.[11]

TABLE 2: Antiepileptic drugs and hormonal contraception interactions

AEDs that lower the effectiveness of oral contraceptives	AEDs that have no effect on oral contraceptives	Estrogen-containing oral contraceptive affecting AEDs levels
Significantly • Carbamazepine • Phenytoin • Phenobarbitone • Oxcarbazepine (dose >1,200 mg) • Clobazam **Weak effect** • Topiramate (dose >200 mg)—induces estrogen only • Lamotrigine—induces progestin only • Felbamate • Rufinamide	• Gabapentin • Levetiracetam • Valproate • Pregabalin • Zonisaimde • Clonazepam • Lacosamide • Ezogabine	**Decreases** • Lamotrigine levels • Valproate levels

AED, antiepileptic drug.

Intramuscular (IM) medroxyprogesterone (Depo-Provera) can be used but the interval between the injections should be reduced to 8–10 weeks rather than the usual 12 weeks. It is associated with weight gain, bone density loss, and delayed return of fertility hence it is not a first-line option.

Emergency Contraception—Is It Safe and Effective?

Postcoital contraception also known as *morning-after pill* is available in the form of two 0.75-mg levonorgestrel pills taken 12 hours apart. The effect of EIAEDs on this levonorgestrel preparation is not known. Royal College of Obstetricians and Gynaecologists recommends giving double dose 12 hours apart (3-mg total dose). Others recommend an initial dose of 1.5 mg followed 12 hours later by an additional 0.75 mg.[12]

WOMEN WITH EPILEPSY AND FERTILITY

Sexual Dysfunction

Nearly 30–40% WWE experience sexual dysfunction. This is manifested as diminished sexual interest and desire, disorders of sexual arousal (dyspareunia, vaginismus, etc.). AEDs may contribute to sexual dysfunction by direct cortical effects or through alterations in the hormonal effect on sexual behavior.[13]

Fertility

Women with epilepsy significantly less fertile than their peer group and this remains true even when adjustments are made for differing marriage rates, etc.[14] The Kerala Registry of Epilepsy and Pregnancy reported a 39% infertility rate among younger women with epilepsy actively trying to conceive after marriage. Again those who were on polytherapy had a 20-fold higher chance of not conceiving.[15] The reasons are unclear although multiple mechanisms have been postulated. Seizures can lead to central dysregulation of the hypothalamic-pituitary ovarian axis, premature ovarian failure and polycystic ovarian syndrome. AEDs alter endogenous hormonal profile thereby decreasing ovulation rates. Apart from biological factors, psychosocial causes and cultural beliefs are the reason that many women with epilepsy choose not to bear children.

Pregnancy and Epilepsy

It is quite challenging to manage epilepsy during pregnancy. Anti-epileptic drugs are among the a few drugs that require continuous use during pregnancy. A vast majority of women with epilepsy are likely to have uneventful pregnancy and healthy baby free of any structural or behavioral abnormality.[16] The pregnancy should not be discouraged in females with epilepsy. Our goal of the treatment is minimal effective doses of medications to avoid any major side effects (including minimal exposure of medicines to the fetus) along with optimal seizure control.

Seizures during Pregnancy

Pregnancy often alters the frequency of epilepsy. About 50% of women report that their epilepsy is better controlled during pregnancy and about 17-37% women report increase in seizures during pregnancy. The increase in seizure frequencies can be attributed to the following factors:

- Poor compliance with prescribed AED, because of the fear of the message that any drug taken during pregnancy can be dangerous to the fetus
- Pregnancy-related fall in plasma drug concentration due to decreased plasma binding, increased drug clearance or increased volume of distribution
- Sleep deprivation
- Hormonal changes
- Stress and anxiety.

Seizures during pregnancy can adversely affect the mother and fetus. Seizures increase the risk of obstetric complications. Recurrent seizures can lead to infants who are small for their gestational age. Also decreased verbal intelligence quotient (IQ) is seen in children, if there are recurrent seizures during gestational period. Generalized seizures increase the risk of premature labor, fetal hypoxemia, infections and even fetal death.[17] In general, women with a 9-12 month baseline of seizure freedom before conception are highly likely to be seizure free throughout pregnancy.

Effects of Anti-epileptic Drugs on Pregnancy

Several international prospective registries have shown almost consistent rates of major structural and cognitive malformations associated with various AEDs. When explaining risks of fetal malformation one should keep in mind that major congenital malformations (MCMs) can occur even in 1-3% healthy women. We should explain that there are more than 90% chances of having a normal pregnancy. The relative risk of major malformation varies with the type of anti-epileptic drug use as well as the dose. Across all registries, valproate has been consistently associated with highest rates of MCMs, ranging from 4.7 to 13.8%.[18] The risk of MCMs is dose dependent for majority of AEDs like carbamazepine, lamotrigine, phenobarbital and valproate. Sodium valproate is having highest risk of teratogenicity especially at doses higher than 1,500 mg per day.[19] Levetiracetam, carbamazepine and lamotrigine are among the safer anti-epileptic drugs from teratogenicity point of view. Phenytoin, phenobarbital and topiramate likely confer an intermediate risk of congenital malformations, whereas data on most other AEDs are too limited to stratify. The majority of these structural abnormalities have already occurred by 8-10 weeks of pregnancy, underscoring the need for early preconception planning.

Polytherapy versus Monotherapy

Malformation rates seen with exposure to carbamazepine or lamotrigine in polytherapy with a drug other than valproate were similar to the rates seen with either drug in monotherapy, whereas if either was combined with valproate, malformation rates were much higher.[20] This suggests that polytherapy regimens that do not include valproate may not increase teratogenic risks as much as previously thought.

Cognitive Teratogenesis

The recent well-designed prospective studies have addressed the issue of cognitive teratogenesis in children exposed to AEDs *in utero*.[21,22] Exposure to valproate was shown to be associated with a decrease in full-scale IQ by approximately 10 points compared to children exposed to other AEDs and control group. This effect was dose related and further increased risk of autism and autism spectrum disorders in exposed children.[22-24] Again, mean IQs were higher in the children of mother who received folate supplementation.

Labor and Delivery

Pregnant-epileptic woman should be referred for the delivery to a center with adult and neonatal intensive care facilities. Ensure regular AED is administered as per the schedule in the early stages of labor [oral/intravenous (IV)]. Risk of developing seizure during labor is 10 times more than during pregnancy. IV lorazepam or IV diazepam has been advocated as the best acute treatment for seizures during labor. Epilepsy by itself is not an indication for cesarean section/induction. Cesarean section is indicated only if seizures occurr during labor.

Principles of Management

Preconception Level

- *Withdrawing drug*—if woman is seizure free for more than 2-4 years and more than 1 year before planning for conception, considering tapering AED [not in cases with Juvenile myoclonic epilepsy/primary generalized epilepsy]
- *Anti-epileptic drug change*—consider AED substitution in patients on relatively more teratogenic drugs like valproate, topiramate and phenobarbital
- *Single drug*—if the woman is on two or more AEDs and well controlled, try to bring down to monotherapy (attempt if more than 1 year preconception; advice about use of contraception during AED changes)
- *Lowest dose*—consider lowering the dose of AED in patients very well controlled on monotherapy
- *Drug level*—establish baseline drug level (ideally trough levels) at least twice before pregnancy.

- *Folic acid*—continue/initiate on folic acid 0.4-4 mg/day along with the AEDs
- *Imaging*—any brain imaging like magnetic resonance imaging if is being considered should ideally be done in this period itself
- *Epilepsy surgery*—in case of drug-resistant epilepsy with surgically remediable substrate.

Periconception and Postconception
- *Continue AEDs*—no AED withdrawals during pregnancy
- Continue folic acid supplementation
- Avoid changes in AEDs unless prompted by poor seizure control
- If available, obtain serum AED levels at regular intervals
    - At 5-6 weeks, at 10 weeks and then at least once each trimester and adjust doses of AED accordingly
    - Repeat in the first or second postpartum week
    - Lamotrigine and levetiracetam may need to be monitored more frequently
- Obtain maternal serum α-fetoprotein or do a triple test at 12-14 weeks
- Targeted anatomic ultrasound ("level II ultrasound") at 18 weeks
- Four-dimensional ultrasonography at 22-24 weeks—for cleft palate, lips and digital anomalies, sensitivity is better
- If patient is on EIAEDs, give vitamin K during the last month and 1 mg administered intramuscularly or intravenously to the newborn at birth
- After delivery—decrease AED dose over 5-10 days to slightly above prepregnancy maintenance dose.

Breastfeeding and Child Care

The benefits of breastfeeding outweighs the theoretical harms of AED exposure via breast milk. Breastfeeding promotes bonding of mother and infant. Breastfeeding reduces risk of infections, diabetes mellitus and sudden infant death syndrome in the infant. Breastfeeding is beneficial for the mother even and it reduces the risk of breast and ovarian cancer as well as diabetes mellitus in the mother. One of the studies found that children exposed to carbamazepine, lamotrigine, phenytoin or valproate in breast milk as infants had higher IQs and language scores at 6 years of age when compared to those children whose mothers were taking AEDs and did not breastfeed.[25] Phenobarbitone and benzodiazepines can cause sedation in the newborn and if seen, mother should be advised to reduce breastfeeds and supplement with bottle-feeds.

Certain precautions in parenting are needed for women with uncontrolled seizures. Patients should avoid bathing their child alone. Do diaper changing on a pad on the floor instead of on a changing table. Consider using a stroller rather than an infant carrier strapped to the mother. The importance of not having an infant sleep in bed with the mother should be stressed.

Bone Health

Women with epilepsy have two- to sixfold higher risks of fractures compared to the general population.[26] Enzyme-inducing AEDs induce cytochrome P450 (CYP) enzyme leading to accelerated metabolism of vitamin D to inactive metabolites and/or lower (free) estradiol levels leading to osteoporosis. Dual-energy X-ray absorptiometry can assess bone mineral density. Those with low T-scores should be treated with calcium and vitamin D supplementation.

CONCLUSION

The effect of female hormones on seizure frequency is important to understand and discuss with patients. Whenever needed intermittent therapy should be instituted for catamenial epilepsy. Given the risk of PCOS, structural and cognitive teratogenesis, valproate is best avoided in a female of childbearing potential. Whenever deemed necessary, valproate should be kept at the lowest dose needed (≤500 mg/day). Barrier or IUDs are the best contraceptive options for WWE. AED optimization and substitution should be done at least more than a year in advance to conception. Preconceptional counseling, folate supplementation, planned pregnancy with careful monitoring and regular follow-up maximize chances for optimal maternal and child outcomes. Breastfeeding should be encouraged and certain precautions are needed while caring for newborn to avoid mishaps. In postmenopausal women with epilepsy on enzyme-inducing AEDs or valproate, it is advised to give calcium and vitamin D supplementation.

REFERENCES

1. Crawford P. Best practice guidelines for the management of women with epilepsy. Epilepsia. 2005;46:117-24.
2. Herzog AG. Catamenial epilepsy: definition, prevalence, pathophysiology and treatment. Seizure. 2008;17:151-9.
3. Herzog AG, Klein P, Ransil BJ. Three patterns of catamenial epilepsy. Epilepsia. 1997;38:1082-8.
4. Foldvary-Schaefer N, Falcone T. Catamenial epilepsy: pathophysiology, diagnosis, and management. Neurology. 2003;61:S2-15.
5. Hart R, Hickey M, Franks S. Definitions, prevalence and symptoms of polycystic ovaries and polycystic ovary syndrome. Best Pract Res Clin Obstet Gynaecol. 2004;18:671-83.
6. Rotterdam ESHRE/ASRM-Sponsored PCOS Consensus Workshop Group. Revised 2003 consensus on diagnostic criteria and long-term health risks related to polycystic ovary syndrome. Fertil Steril. 2004;81:19-25.
7. Sahota P, Prabhakar S, Kharbanda PS, Bhansali A, Jain V, Das CP, et al. Seizure type, antiepileptic drugs, and reproductive endocrine dysfunction in Indian women with epilepsy: a cross-sectional study. Epilepsia. 2008;49:2069-77.
8. Herzog AG, Schachter SC. On the association between valproate and polycystic ovary syndrome. Epilepsia. 2001;42:311-5.

9. Davis AR, Pack AM, Kritzer J, Yoon A, Camus A. Reproductive history, sexual behavior and use of contraception in women with epilepsy. Contraception. 2008;77:405-9.
10. Gaffield ME, Culwell KR, Lee CR. The use of hormonal contraception among women taking anticonvulsant therapy. Contraception. 2011;83:16-29.
11. Bounds W, Guillebaud J. Observational series on women using the contraceptive Mirena concurrently with anti-epileptic and other enzyme-inducing drugs. J Fam Plann Reprod Health Care. 2002;28:78-80.
12. Schwenkhagen AM, Stodieck SR. Which contraception for women with epilepsy? Seizure. 2008;17:145-50.
13. Morrell MJ, Flynn KL, Doñe S, Flaster E, Kalayjian L, Pack AM. Sexual dysfunction, sex steroid hormone abnormalities, and depression in women with epilepsy treated with antiepileptic drugs. Epilepsy Behav. 2005;6:360-5.
14. Thomas SV, Deetha TD, Kurup JR, Reghunath B, Radhakrishnan K, Sarma PS. Pregnancy among women with epilepsy. Ann Indian Acad Neurology. 1999;2:123-8.
15. Sukumaran SC, Sarma PS, Thomas SV. Polytherapy increases the risk of infertility in women with epilepsy. Neurology. 2010;75:1351-5.
16. Hill DS, Wlodarczyk BJ, Palacios AM, Finnell RH. Teratogenic effects of antiepileptic drugs. Expert Rev Neurother. 2010;10:943-59.
17. Sveberg L, Svalheim S, Taubøll E. The impact of seizures on pregnancy and delivery. Seizure. 2015;28:35-8.
18. Tomson T, Xue H, Battino D. Major congenital malformations in children of women with epilepsy. Seizure. 2015;28:40-4.
19. Meador KJ, Loring DW. Developmental effects of antiepileptic drugs and the need for improved regulations. Neurology. 2016;86:297-306.
20. Holmes LB, Mittendorf R, Shen A, Smith CR, Hernandez-Diaz S. Fetal effects of anticonvulsant polytherapies: different risks from different drug combinations. Arch Neurol. 2011;68:1275-81.
21. Meador KJ, Baker GA, Browning N, Cohen MJ, Bromley RL, Clayton-Smith J, et al. Fetal antiepileptic drug exposure and cognitive outcomes at age 6 years (NEAD study): a prospective observational study. Lancet Neurol. 2013;12:244-52.
22. Baker GA, Bromley RL, Briggs M, Cheyne CP, Cohen MJ, García-Fiñana M, et al. IQ at 6 years following in utero exposure to antiepileptic drugs: a controlled cohort study. Neurology. 2015;84:382-90.
23. Christensen J, Grønborg TK, Sørensen MJ, Schendel D, Parner ET, Pedersen LH, et al. Prenatal valproate exposure and risk of autism spectrum disorders and childhood autism. JAMA. 2013;309:1696-1703.
24. Wood AG, Nadebaum C, Anderson V, Reutens D, Barton S, O>Brien TJ, et al. Prospective assessment of autism traits in children exposed to antiepileptic drugs during pregnancy. Epilepsia 2015;56:1047-55.
25. Meador KJ, Baker GA, Browning N, Cohen MJ, Bromley RL, Clayton-Smith J, et al. Breastfeeding in children of women taking antiepileptic drugs: cognitive outcomes at age 6 years. JAMA Pediatr. 2014;168:729-36.
26. Brodie MJ, Mintzer S, Pack AM, Gidal BE, Vecht CJ, Schmidt D. Enzyme induction with antiepileptic drugs: cause for concern? Epilepsia. 2013;54:11-27.

CHAPTER 8

Drug-resistant Epilepsy

Rajesh Shankar Iyer

INTRODUCTION

Epilepsy accounts for 1% of global disease burden, which is equivalent to lung cancer in men and breast cancer in women.[1] Ten percent of the world's population will have at least one seizure during their lifetime whereas 1% has active epilepsy.[2] Around 30–40% of people with epilepsy fail to get adequate control of their seizures with anti-epileptic drugs (AEDs).[3] These patients are classified as having drug-resistant epilepsy (DRE). The diagnosis of DRE carries with it a poor prognostic implication and a compromised quality-of-life (QOL). In this chapter, we try to understand the etiology, mechanisms, complications and comorbidities and management of DRE.

DEFINITION

A formal consensus definition of DRE was proposed by an Ad Hoc Task Force of the International League against Epilepsy (ILAE) in 2010. It defined DRE as the failure of adequate trials of two tolerated, appropriately chosen and used AED schedules (whether as monotherapies or in combination) to achieve sustained seizure freedom.[4]

PREDICTORS OF DRUG RESISTANCE

The response to the first AED is a powerful prognostic indicator of refractoriness. Kwan and Brodie in their landmark study found that only 11% of those who did not respond to the first drug subsequently became seizure free.[5] On adding the second drug, only 3% became seizure free. Studies have shown that the presence of a neurologic deficit at the onset of the disease, magnetic resonance imaging (MRI) defined underlying structural abnormality, presence of developmental delay and high frequency of seizures at the disease onset are consistent predictors of DRE.[6-10] A syndromic approach (Chapter 2) to epilepsies is highly useful in this regard as symptomatic epilepsies are more drug-resistant compared to the idiopathic ones. Drug resistance is more often the rule than exception in some well-defined pediatric epilepsy syndromes, such as neonatal Ohtahara Syndrome, West syndrome, severe myoclonic epilepsy of infancy (SMEI or Dravet's syndrome), myoclonic-astatic epilepsy (MAE or Doose syndrome), Lennox-Gastaut syndrome (LGS), Rasmussen encephalitis and partial epilepsies associated with cortical dysplasias.

MECHANISMS OF DRUG RESISTANCE

The exact mechanism of DRE is not known and is considered multifactorial. The currently hypothesized biologic mechanisms of DRE operate at three molecular locations.[11]

Failure of Drugs to Reach their Targets

This transporter or pharmacokinetic hypothesis proposes that DRE may be due to overexpression of multidrug efflux transporters like P-glycoprotein in the capillary endothelial cells. They maintain the integrity of blood-brain barrier and reduce accumulation of drugs in the brain by pumping them from the intracellular space back into the capillary lumen. Polymorphisms of the gene encoding P-glycoprotein (ABCB1) may be associated with DRE.[12]

Alteration of Targets

This target or pharmacodynamic hypothesis postulates that response to drugs is reduced by alteration in the cellular targets. For example:
- Polymorphisms of the *SCN2A* gene may lead to resistance to AEDs acting on the sodium channels[13]
- Gamma-aminobutyric acid type-A (GABA$_A$) receptor subtypes have shown altered expression in people with drug-resistant temporal lobe epilepsy.[14]

Missing the Real Targets

Autoantibodies to ion channels including voltage-gated potassium and calcium channels, glutamate N-methyl-D-aspartate (NMDA) and γ-aminobutyric acid type-B (GABA$_B$) receptors have been found pathogenic in patients with autoimmune epilepsies.[15-17] They do not respond to AEDs and more often respond to immunotherapies.[18] Similarly, other mechanisms of epileptogenesis not affected by conventional AEDs include mitochondrial oxidative stress and electrical coupling in gap junctions in neurons and glial cells.[19,20]

PSEUDORESISTANCE

Before confirming DRE, "pseudoresistance" resulting from inadequate and inappropriate treatment of the underlying disorder must be ruled out. The following situations are responsible for this phenomenon:

- Wrong diagnosis: The various mimics as discussed in Chapter 3 should be ruled out before entertaining a diagnosis of epilepsy. Common mimickers are vasovagal syncope, cardiac arrhythmias, metabolic disturbances, transient ischemic attacks and migraine. More than 25% of apparently DRE in adults turns out to be psychogenic nonepileptic seizures[21]
- Wrong drugs: Treatment failure and sometimes seizure aggravation can occur with incorrect classification of seizure types and syndromes. The latest trends in classification of seizures and syndromes are outlined in Chapter 2. Carbamazepine, oxcarbazepine, phenytoin, vigabatrin and gabapentin can worsen absence epilepsy and myoclonic seizures.[22] Polypharmacy with inappropriate drug combinations due to lack of understanding of their pharmacokinetic properties is another reason for treatment failure
- Wrong dose: Suboptimal dosage of AEDs especially due to over-reliance on the therapeutic drug levels than the clinical situation can also lead to pseudoresistance
- Wrong life style: Lack of adherence to treatment schedule and missing doses, alcohol and drug abuse, sleep deprivation and stress are also responsible for apparent treatment failure.

CONSEQUENCES OF DRUG RESISTANCE

Disease Progression

The concept that "seizures beget seizures" was introduced by William Gowers in 1881.[23] This concept is a bit controversial at the moment with evidences both for and against it. Progressive brain damage over time has been demonstrated in serial neuroimaging studies especially in relation to temporal lobe epilepsy.[24-28] Recurrent seizures due to a primary seizure focus can lead to the development of an independent secondary focus. This phenomenon of secondary epileptogenesis has been demonstrated in animals by kindling studies.[29,30] In humans, spikes from the opposite temporal lobe present before surgery have been shown to disappear after successful temporal lobe surgery.[31]

Mortality and Morbidity

There seems to be a 1.6–11.4 times greater mortality risk in people with epilepsy.[32] This is more so with symptomatic epilepsies and less with idiopathic epilepsies.[33] Death can happen due to traffic accidents, drowning, burns and work place injuries. Death as a direct consequence of epilepsy can happen due to status epilepticus or sudden unexpected death in epilepsy (SUDEP). SUDEP is defined as "sudden, unexpected, witnessed or unwitnessed, nontraumatic and nondrowning death occurring in benign circumstances, in an individual with epilepsy, with or without evidence of a preceding seizure and excluding documented status epilepticus".[34] SUDEP occurs in 1 per 1,000 patients with epilepsy per year and in 6 per 1,000 patients with DRE per year.[35] It is thus more common in people with uncontrolled seizures, especially in those with convulsive and nocturnal seizures.[36,37] Controlling seizures is the only effective method of decreasing SUDEP. People who are seizure free after epilepsy surgery enjoy the benefit of a markedly reduced risk of SUDEP.[38,39]

Anti-epileptic Drugs-related Side Effects

This is discussed in detail in Chapter 6. The side effects in general can be dose related, hypersensitivity reactions, effects due to long-term use, drug-drug interactions related to the use of first generation AEDs, metabolic side effects related to P450-inducing drugs and cognitive teratogenicity.

Neuropsychiatric Disturbances

Neuropsychiatric comorbidities are seen in around 50–60% of people with epilepsy. Many of these comorbidities are coexistent and are unlikely to be directly caused by seizures. However, some of them like anxiety and mood disorders including depression and memory and cognitive disturbances could also be the result of recurrent seizures or the continuous use of AEDs.

MANAGEMENT

Various treatment options as discussed below are available while dealing with DRE. However, a personalized treatment plan based on the patient's cultural and socioeconomic conditions should be formulated and followed.

Rule Out Pseudoresistance

One must be absolutely sure that it is DRE and not any of the mimics. In case of doubt, video monitoring and recording of events should be done for confirmation of diagnosis.

Newer Anti-epileptic Drugs

They are produced either as modification of the already available AEDs or with novel mechanisms of action and may be tried in DRE.
- Modification of parent AED:
    - Fluorofelbamate: An analog of felbamate without adverse effects like aplastic anemia and hepatic failure and hence better safety

- Eslicarbazepine: Better tolerability than oxcarbazepine or carbamazepine
- Pregabalin: Greater binding to voltage-gated calcium channels compared to gabapentin and hence more efficacy
- Novel action:
    - Rufinamide: Acts by limiting high-frequency firing of sodium-dependent action potentials useful in LGS[40,41]
    - Stiripentol: For the treatment of Dravet's syndrome[42]
    - Retigabine: Unique action as potassium channel opener and used as add-on for refractory partial seizures in adults[43]
    - Brivaracetam: Binds to the synaptic vesicle protein-2A molecule
    - Perampanel: Modulates glutamate neurotransmission mediated by α-amino-3-hydroxy-5-methyl-4-isoxazolepropionic acid (AMPA).[44]
    - Ganaxolone: Neuroactive steroid with $GABA_A$ receptor modulator effect and found useful in infantile spasms.[45]

Rational Combination of Anti-epileptic Drugs

When one AED fails to control seizures, rational polypharmacy may be tried. This would generally mean combining AEDs with different modes of action rather than those with similar mechanisms. This helps in benefitting out of synergistic effects of the drugs and avoids the neurotoxic effects due to use of similarly acting drugs. Examples of good polypharmacy would include sodium valproate and lamotrigine, carbamazepine or phenytoin with phenobarbitone or clobazam. Similarly the combination of phenytoin and carbamazepine is best avoided since both are sodium channel blockers.

Resective Epilepsy Surgery

Patients with DRE should be evaluated early for epilepsy surgery. Those with surgically remediable, epilepsy syndromes should be identified and subjected to surgery at the earliest. The various surgical procedures and approaches have been detailed in Chapter 10. The various surgically remediable epilepsy syndromes are:
- Mesial temporal lobe atrophy associated with hippocampal sclerosis (MTLE-HS)
- Focal structural lesions. For example, focal cortical dysplasias and developmental tumors
- Diffuse hemispherical lesions:
    - Hemimegalencephaly
    - Rasmussen encephalitis
    - Sturge-Weber syndrome
    - Childhood insults resulting in unihemispherical lesions like gliosis, infarcts and porencephalic cysts
- Gelastic seizures associated with hypothalamic hamartomas.

Palliative Epilepsy Surgery

Palliative surgeries are considered when resective surgeries are not possible. They disrupt pathways of epileptiform discharges and can help in reduction in the frequency and severity of seizures.
- Corpus callosotomy: Disconnection procedure done in children with symptomatic generalized epilepsy and severe intellectual disability like LGS. They are particularly useful in reducing the atonic seizures causing drop attacks and injuries
- Multiple subpial transections: This is done when resective surgery is not possible due to the close proximity of the lesion to the eloquent cortex
- Stereotactic techniques: They are done in people who have medical comorbidities making them unfit for open surgeries. Gamma knife surgery is a form of noninvasive stereotactic radiotherapy.[46] Its benefits take months or years to show. A laser-ablative approach using an intracranial probe gives immediate results.[47]

Neurostimulation

Vagus Nerve Stimulation

This involves implantation of a device, which delivers regular electrical impulses to the vagus nerve. This is done by an extracranial procedure wherein a generator is implanted into a pouch beneath the left clavicle. The leads of the vagus nerve stimulation (VNS) device are wrapped around the left vagus nerve by an incision in the neck and the electrodes are connected to the generator. Vagal nerve stimulation modulates seizure control and has a positive impact on mood probably by altering norepinephrine release by projections of the solitary tract to the locus coeruleus, increasing GABA levels and inhibiting aberrant cortical activity by the reticular-activating system. Seizure freedom after VNS is a rarity and on an average 50% of patients gets 50% reduction in seizures.[48]

Deep Brain Stimulation

This is tried using intracranial electrodes to stimulate various subcortical structures including subthalamic and caudate nuclei, anterior and centromedian thalamic nuclei, the cerebellum and the hippocampus.[49] The aim of deep brain stimulation (DBS) is to set the brain to its preseizure status and prevent its re-entry into a seizure-producing mode.

Responsive Nerve Stimulation

Here, subdural and intraparenchymal electrodes are used in a closed-loop fashion. The implanted electrodes detect the seizure onset. They send an electrical stimulation to the seizure focus, which would abort the seizures.[50]

Trigeminal Nerve Stimulation

Here, electrodes are applied to the skin of the forehead intermittently and electrical signals are delivered to the branches of trigeminal nerve which in turn would modulate selected brain regions including the nucleus solitarius, the locus coeruleus, the vagus nerve and the cerebral cortex.[51]

Ketogenic Diet

The ketogenic diet is a high-fat, low-protein and low-carbohydrate diet. It is used mainly in children with DRE. Nonadherence is a major issue due to the unpleasant dietary regimen.

Alternative Therapies

Homeopathy, acupuncture, psychological techniques and herbal treatments are often used though none have been proven to be definitely useful. On the contrary, some can cause adverse effects by interacting with AEDs, e.g., *Gingkgo biloba* can lower serum concentrations of phenytoin and sodium valproate.[52] However, behavioral therapeutic approaches can recognize and avoid seizure triggers and are useful in reflex epilepsies.[53] Stress reduction by meditation can probably have a beneficial effect on seizure occurrence.

CONCLUSION

Despite the introduction of many AEDs, approximately one-thirds of people with epilepsy remain drug-resistant. Managing DRE is highly challenging and requires a multidisciplinary approach. The consequences of DRE are many and affect the individual's QOL. DRE should be identified early to try and prevent or minimize these consequences. Pseudoresistance should be considered and ruled out. Resective surgery, for the eligible candidate remains the treatment of choice for DRE. The treating physician should look for the possibility of surgical treatment and refer to specialized centers for evaluating DRE. The classical description of a complex partial seizure of temporal onset, the presence of an infantile hemiplegia or the presence of tonic head drops with scars are clues for the busy physician to suspect surgical candidacy. Similarly, any imaging findings of developmental lesions or mesial temporal sclerosis should alert the clinician of surgical possibility. An individualized approach in selecting the other options is warranted, if surgery is not feasible. Despite all our efforts a good number of patients would still get repetitive seizures necessitating supportive care. More and more research to unravel the mystery of DRE needs to be undertaken for a much more effective management of the unfortunate patient.

REFERENCES

1. Murray CJ, Lopez AD. Global Comparative Assessment in the Health Sector; Disease Burden, Expenditures, and Intervention Packages. Geneva: World Health Organization; 1994.
2. Hesdorffer DC, Logroscino G, Benn EK, Katri N, Cascino G, Hauser WA. Estimating risk for developing epilepsy: A population based study in Rochester, Minnesota. Neurology. 2011;76:23-7.
3. Kobau R, Zahran H, Thurman DJ, Zack MM, Henry TR, Schachter SC, et al. Centers for Disease Control and Prevention (CDC). Epilepsy surveillance among adults19 states, Behavioral Risk Factor Surveillance System, 2005. MMWR Surveill Summ. 2008;57:1-20.
4. Kwan P, Arzimanoglou A, Berg AT, Brodie MJ, Allen Hauser W, Mathern G, et al. Definition of drug resistant epilepsy: consensus proposal by the ad hoc Task Force of the ILAE Commission on Therapeutic Strategies. Epilepsia. 2010;51:1069-77.
5. Kwan P, Brodie MJ. Early identification of refractory epilepsy. N Engl J Med. 2000;342:314-9.
6. Sillanpää M, Schmidt D. Is incident drug-resistance of childhood-onset epilepsy reversible? A long-term follow-up study. Brain. 2012;135:2256-62.
7. Semah F, Picot MC, Adam C, Broglin D, Arzimanoglou A, Bazin B, et al. Is the underlying cause of epilepsy a major prognostic factor for recurrence? Neurology. 1998;51:1256-62.
8. Trinka E, Martin F, Luef G, Unterberger I, Bauer G. Chronic epilepsy with complex partial seizures is not always medically intractable—a long-term observational study. Acta Neurol Scand. 2001;103:219-25.
9. Wirrell E, Wong-Kisiel L, Mandrekar J, Nickels K. Predictors and course of medically intractable epilepsy in young children presenting before 36 months of age: a retrospective, population-based study. Epilepsia. 2012;53:1563-9.
10. Seker YB, Okuyaz C, Komur M. Predictors of intractable childhood epilepsy. Pediatr Neurol. 2013;48:52-5.
11. Kwan P, Schachter SC, Brodie MJ. Drug-resistant epilepsy. N Engl J Med. 2011;365:919-26.
12. Siddiqui A, Kerb R, Weale ME, Brinkmann U, Smith A, Goldstein DB, et al. Association of multidrug resistance in epilepsy with a polymorphism in the drug transporter gene ABCB1. N Engl J Med. 2003;348:1442-8.
13. Kwan P, Poon WS, Ng HK, Kang DE, Wong V, Ng PW, et al. Multidrug resistance in epilepsy and polymorphisms in the voltage-gated sodium channel genes SCN1A, SCN2A, and SCN3A: correlation among phenotype, genotype, and mRNA expression. Pharmacogenet Genomics. 2008;18:989-98.
14. Loup F, Picard F, Yonekawa Y, Wieser HG, Fritschy JM. Selective changes in GABAA receptor subtypes in white matter neurons of patients with focal epilepsy. Brain. 2009;132:2449-63.
15. McKnight K, Jiang Y, Hart Y, Cavey A, Wroe S, Blank M, et al. Serum antibodies in epilepsy and seizure associated disorders. Neurology. 2005;65:1730-6.
16. Dalmau J, Gleichman AJ, Hughes EG, Rossi JE, Peng X, Lai M, et al. Anti-NMDA-receptor encephalitis: case series and analysis of the effects of antibodies. Lancet Neurol. 2008;7:1091-8.
17. Lancaster E, Lai M, Peng X, Hughes E, Constantinescu R, Raizer J, et al. Antibodies to the GABA(B) receptor in limbic encephalitis with seizures: case series and characterisation of the antigen. Lancet Neurol. 2010;9:67-76.
18. Vincent A, Irani SR, Lang B. The growing recognition of immunotherapy responsive seizure disorders with autoantibodies to specific neuronal proteins. Curr Opin Neurol. 2010;23:144-50.

19. Waldbaum S, Patel M. Mitochondria, oxidative stress, and temporal lobe epilepsy. Epilepsy Res. 2010;88:23-45.
20. Voss LJ, Jacobson G, Sleigh JW, Steyn-Ross A, Steyn-Ross M. Excitatory effects of gap junction blockers on cerebral cortex seizure-like activity in rats and mice. Epilepsia. 2009;50:1971-8.
21. Smith D, Defalla BA, Chadwick DW. The misdiagnosis of epilepsy and the management of refractory epilepsy in a specialist clinic. QJM. 1999;92:15-23.
22. Menon R, Baheti NN, Cherian A, Iyer RS. Oxcarbazepine induced worsening of seizures in Jeavons syndrome: lessons learnt from an interesting presentation. Neurol India. 2011;59:70-2.
23. Gowers WR. Epilepsy and other chronic convulsive disorders: their causes, symptoms and treatment. London: J&A Churchill; 1881.
24. Fuerst D, Shah J, Shah A, Watson C. Hippocampal sclerosis is a progressive disorder: a longitudinal volumetric MRI study. Ann Neurol. 2003;53:413-6.
25. Cendes F. Progressive hippocampal and extrahippocampal atrophy in drug resistant epilepsy. Curr Opin Neurol. 2005;18:173-7.
26. Briellmann RS, Berkovic SF, Syngeniotis A, King MA, Jackson GD. Seizure-associated hippocampal volume loss: a longitudinal magnetic resonance study of temporal lobe epilepsy. Ann Neurol. 2002;51:641-4.
27. Bernhardt BC, Worsley KJ, Kim H, Evans AC, Bernasconi A, Bernasconi N. Longitudinal and cross-sectional analysis of atrophy in pharmacoresistant temporal lobe epilepsy. Neurology. 2009;72:1747-54.
28. Bonilha L, Rorden C, Appenzeller S, Coan AC, Cendes F, Li LM. Gray matter atrophy associated with duration of temporal lobe epilepsy. Neuroimage. 2006;32:1070-9.
29. Sato M, Nakashima T. Kindling: secondary epileptogenesis, sleep and catecholamines. Can J Neurol Sci. 1975;2:439-46.
30. Morrell F. Secondary epileptogenesis in man. Arch Neurol. 1985;42:318-35.
31. Patrick S, Berg A, Spencer SS. EEG and seizure outcome after epilepsy surgery. Epilepsia. 1995;36:236-40.
32. Holst AG, Winkel BG, Risgaard B, Nielsen JB, Rasmussen PV, Haunsø S, et al. Epilepsy and risk of death and sudden unexpected death in the young: a nationwide study. Epilepsia. 2013;54:1613-20.
33. Gaitatzis A, Johnson AL, Chadwick DW, Shorvon SD, Sander JW. Life expectancy in people with newly diagnosed epilepsy. Brain. 2004;127:2427-32.
34. Nashef L, So EL, Ryvlin P, Tomson T. Unifying the definitions of sudden unexpected death in epilepsy. Epilepsia. 2012;53:227-33.
35. Thurman DJ. The epidemiology of SUDEP: a public health perspective. Epilepsy Curr. 2013;13:9.
36. Shorvon S, Tomson T. Sudden unexpected death in epilepsy. Lancet. 2011;378:2028-38.
37. Devinsky O. Sudden, unexpected death in epilepsy. N Engl J Med. 2011;365:1801-11.
38. Bell GS, Sinha S, Tisi JD, Stephani C, Scott CA, Harkness WF, et al. Premature mortality in refractory partial epilepsy: Does surgical treatment make a difference? J Neurol Neurosurg Psychiatry. 2010;81:716-8.
39. Jehi L. Sudden death in epilepsy, surgery, and seizure outcomes: the interface between heart and brain. Cleve Clin J Med. 2010;77:S51-5.
40. Hakimian S, Cheng-Hakimian A, Anderson GD, Miller JW. Rufinamide: a new antiepileptic medication. Expert Opin Pharmacother. 2007;8:1931-40.
41. Glauser T, Kluger G, Sachdeo R, Krauss G, Perdomo C, Arroyo S. Rufinamide for generalized seizures associated with Lennox-Gastaut syndrome. Neurology. 2008;70:1950-8.
42. Chiron C. Stiripentol. Neurotherapeutics. 2007;4:123-5.

43. Brodie MJ, Lerche H, Gil-Nagel A, Elger C, Hall S, Shin P, et al. Efficacy and safety of adjunctive ezogabine (retigabine) in refractory partial epilepsy. Neurology. 2010;75:1817-24.
44. Bialer M, White HS. Key factors in the discovery and development of new antiepileptic drugs. Nat Rev Drug Discov. 2010;9:68-82.
45. Kerrigan JF, Shields WD, Nelson TY, Bluestone DL, Dodson WE, Bourgeois BF, et al. Ganaxolone for treating intractable infantile spasms: a multicenter, open-label, add-on trial. Epilepsy Res. 2000;42:133-9.
46. Quigg M, Ralston J, Barbaro N. Radiosurgery for epilepsy: Clinical experience and potential antiepileptic mechanisms. Epilepsia. 2012;53:7-15.
47. Curry DJ, Gowda A, McNichols RJ, Wilfong AA. MR-guided stereotactic laser ablation of epileptogenic foci in children. Epilepsy Behav. 2012;24:408-14.
48. Schachter SC, Boon P. Vagus nerve stimulation. In: Engel J Jr, Pedley TA (Eds). Epilepsy: A Comprehensive Textbook, 2nd edition. Philadelphia: Lippincott Raven; 2008. pp. 1395-9.
49. Fisher R, Salanova V, Witt T, Worth R, Henry T, Gross R, et al. The SANTE Study Group. Electrical stimulation of the anterior nucleus of thalamus for treatment of refractory epilepsy. Epilepsia. 2010;51:899-908.
50. Morrell MJ. RNS System in Epilepsy Study Group. Responsive cortical stimulation for the treatment of medically intractable partial epilepsy. Neurology. 2011;77:1295-304.
51. DeGiorgio CM, Soss J, Cook IA, Markovic D, Gornbein J, Murray D, et al. Randomized controlled trial of trigeminal nerve stimulation for drug resistant epilepsy. Neurology. 2013;80:786-91.
52. Kupiec T, Raj V. Fatal seizures due to potential herb-drug interactions with Ginkgo biloba. J Anal Toxicol. 2005;29:755-8.
53. Michaelis R, Schonfeld W, Elsas SM. Trigger self-control and seizure arrest in the Andrews/Reiter behavioral approach to epilepsy: A retrospective analysis of seizure frequency. Epilepsy Behav. 2012;23:266-71.

CHAPTER 9

Status Epilepticus: The Current Status

Ramshekhar N Menon, Ashalatha Radhakrishnan

INTRODUCTION

The term status epilepticus (SE) is used to describe a state of recurrent or uninterrupted seizures, which impede normal brain function. If this medical emergency is left untreated, it results in high morbidity and mortality.[1-3] Status epilepticus has an overall annual incidence of 10–41 per 100,000.[1-6] Age-specific incidence rates are indicative of a U-shaped curve with peaks in the pediatric and elderly age groups.[7] Mortality and morbidity rates of SE are determined by the underlying etiology, patients age, and convulsive versus nonconvulsive seizure types. Due to multiple deterministic factors, fatality rates in different studies are quite heterogeneous ranging from 3 to 33%.[1-3]

DEFINITION AND CLASSIFICATION

Status epilepticus is defined as "a seizure that persists for a sufficient length of time, or repeated frequently enough that recovery between attacks does not occur".[8] Considering methodological and operational differences between studies, definitions and classifications keep evolving.[9] In this chapter, SE is classified based on the persistence or absence of overt motor manifestations into convulsive and nonconvulsive.[10]

Convulsive Status Epilepticus

This entity is characterized by generalized tonic-clonic SE and is the most deleterious type of SE. This is recognized when generalized convulsive seizure activity recurs with incomplete recovery of sensorium between seizures or as a single prolonged convulsion.[11] As mentioned previously, controversies related to the definition of duration of convulsive SE abound. Most studies have suggested convulsive activity lasting at least 30 minutes for defining SE based on experimental evidence of irreversible neuronal damage after about half an hour of continuing epileptic activity, which can become self-sustaining.[12] However, with evidence from clinical data, which indicates that spontaneous cessation of generalized convulsive seizures is unlikely after 5 minutes, a duration of 5 minutes as proposed by Lowenstein et al. is considered practical for adults and children aged above 5 years as it mandates recognition of an impending medical emergency.[11]

Nonconvulsive Status Epilepticus

Nonconvulsive status epilepticus (NCSE) is a term designated to indicate ongoing electromechanical dissociation congruent to ongoing dynamically evolving or rhythmic epileptiform discharges on electroencephalography (EEG) without discernible motor phenomenology or overt clinical manifestations other than an altered mental status or coma.[13] Previously, the term subtle SE was used to indicate a persistent encephalopathy accompanied by clinical manifestations as a continuum of convulsive SE. Two subtypes of NCSE are recognized: (i) absence SE which is seen in primary generalized epilepsies or in epileptic encephalopathies such as Lennox-Gastaut syndrome and (ii) complex partial SE which has etiologies similar to convulsive SE in addition to unique syndromes with chromosomal aberrations. Management of NCSE is similar to convulsive SE utilizing EEG, rather than the often indiscernible clinical features alone as a determinant of therapeutic response. Some cases of complex partial SE evolve into generalized NCSE. In other cases, treatment with benzodiazepines and initiation or adjustment in the dose of other anti-epileptic drugs (AEDs) may avoid generalization and the need for intravenous (IV) anesthesia. The degree of obtundation/coma should guide the aggressiveness of therapy in complex partial SE. Comatose NCSE is a relatively newer term to indicate coma accompanied by continuous or periodic epileptiform discharges on EEG with or without minor motor activity and is largely reflective of the underlying etiology of coma.[13] Aggressive AED therapy alone in this situation may not lead to a consistent response in patients unless the causative disorder is addressed.

PATHOPHYSIOLOGICAL PHASES OF STATUS EPILEPTICUS

Pathophysiological evolution of SE commences with a compensated stage wherein physiologic mechanisms prevent cerebral injury and contribute to the metabolic load due to seizures. Following 0.5–1 hour of continuous seizures, a second or the decompensated stage commences wherein this compensation is undermined and subsequently mediates neuronal injury.[12,14] This phase may be potentiated and enhanced by hypotension, hypoxia, hypoglycemia, acidosis, and raised intracranial pressure. The direct cytotoxic effects of seizure discharges are evidenced by periictal imaging findings such as laminar necrosis, which is, however, reversible. Similar characteristics that render susceptibility of neurons to necrosis also predispose these to metabolic and perfusion-based supply-demand mismatch. This is indicative of a neuroprotective window as seen in stroke pathophysiology. Beyond this window, excitotoxic mechanisms result in opening of calcium channels and glutamate-mediated neuronal injury leading to an event cascade that is responsible for necrosis and apoptosis with oxidative stress. Conceptualization of these mechanisms is crucial to the urgency in timing therapeutic interventions in SE and is responsible for the clinical stages discussed below.

Clinical Staging of Status Epilepticus

With the time-dependent evolution of medical refractoriness and development of neuronal injury in SE, prudence dictates the physician to intervene prior to the established self-sustaining phase. Most intervention strategies are planned in accordance with the stages mentioned below.[15]

Impending or Developing Status Epilecticus

As mentioned previously, the presence of continuous or intermittent seizures lasting more than 5 minutes without full recovery of consciousness between the seizures is indicative of this stage. Literature supports this time-based framework as duration of a single seizure is not found to exceed 2 minutes and a cutoff of 5 minutes is 18 standard deviations from the mean duration.[16] In another study, though less than half the seizures lasting between 10 and 30 minutes were shown to cease spontaneously without treatment. Thus, all seizures persisting beyond a 5 minute mark may not evolve into established SE, but ought to be considered as a predictive risk factor.[17] In a controlled environment, an urgent EEG is indicated in the following situations:
- If a patient remains unresponsive for 30 minutes or longer after treatment for a generalized tonic-clonic or complex partial SE
- In any patient who remains poorly responsive in conditions at high risk of seizures, e.g., post-neurosurgery including post-trauma or acute brain insults such as major hemispheric cerebrovascular accidents
- Patients found comatose with no alternative explanation.

Established Status Epilepticus

A situation, wherein clinical or electrographic seizures last beyond 30 minutes with incomplete recovery of consciousness between the episodes. This is supported by experimental evidence of self-sustenance of seizure activity beyond this time-window resulting in distinct seizure-induced neuronal injury as well as pharmacoresistance.[18]

Refractory Status Epilepticus

Status epilepticus becomes refractory when seizures persist despite optimal initial first- and second-line intervention levels, and typically, this stage requires treatment with anesthetic agents. About 12–43% of cases of SE become refractory.[19,20] The majority of cases begin with generalized convulsive SE and 40% of these become nonconvulsive by the time anesthetic agents are initiated. Episodes of refractory status epilepticus (RSE), that develop in the absence of a history, of epilepsy are usually the result of an acute brain injury or drug intoxication or withdrawal.

Subtle Status Epilepticus

Following prolonged generalized convulsive SE or after its active treatment, subtle motor or electroencephalographic activity may persist with continuing neuronal injury. This warrants continuation of aggressive management.[21] This may be considered to be a form of proper NCSE.

STATUS EPILEPTICUS PATHOPHYSIOLOGY

Animal models demonstrate a tendency for self-sustenance of recurrent clinical and electrographic seizures irrespective of the removal of a precipitating stimulus or insult on the mature brain. Drugs that augment inhibition or reduce excitation of the nerve membrane potential are beneficial in the initial phases of convulsive SE.[18,22] In the scenario of established SE, limited agents are efficacious, especially those with novel mechanisms such as those with act via inhibition of the glutamatergic transport or opening of potassium channels.[22] Drugs acting via potentiation of γ-aminobutyric acid (GABA)-ergic transmission demonstrate 20-fold reduction in efficacy following half an hour of persistent seizure activity.[23] Changes in protein phosphorylation constitute one of the basic pathophysiological molecular mechanisms, which operate during SE. As a consequence, alteration in receptor-signaling pathways involving neurotransmitters and modulation of neuronal plasticity occur via changes in protein expression. This may lead to externalization or internalization of the receptors and as a result reduction in the GABA receptor subunits and increase in expressivity of the N-methyl-D-aspartate (NMDA) glutamate receptor subunits on the membrane surface. Acute and overt downregulation of adenosine A1 activity may contribute to excitability of the neuronal membrane. Genetic mechanisms have an uncertain role due to epigenetic modifiers partly annulled by the inhibition of protein synthesis. Predominantly inhibitory neuropeptides like dynorphin, galanin, somatostatin, and neuropeptide Y are depleted in the hippocampus, whereas the relative expression of the proconvulsant tachykinins, substance P, and neurokinin B is elevated. Status epilepticus mediates neuronal loss, which continues to occur despite the absence of motor manifestations due to indolent excitotoxic mechanisms, which cause cellular apoptosis.[24,25]

Etiology

Etiological classification of SE is as follows:
- Acute symptomatic: Causative acute medical or neurological illness
- Remote symptomatic: Remote insults including to formation of gliotic cerebral scar tissue, e.g., an antecedent insult such as meningo-encephalitis, perinatal insult, stroke, or calcified granuloma
- Cryptogenic: SE presumed to be symptomatic, but the cause is unclear and may have a genetic basis or occurs *de novo*
- Status epilepticus in established focal and generalized epilepsy syndromes.

These are summarized in table 1. Remote symptomatic causes, such as cerebrovascular disease, constitute the predominant etiology in developed countries, whereas in developing countries, acute symptomatic causes, such as central nervous system (CNS) infections, account for the majority, varying between 20 and 67% in various studies.[26-33] A prospective study from India highlighted that the etiology was acute symptomatic in 54% (with CNS infections such as neurocysticercosis, encephalitis, or meningoencephalitis predominating), remote symptomatic in 7%, and cryptogenic in 19%. In one-fifth of patients, breakthrough SE secondary to poor AED compliance was identified.[33] New onset refractory status epilepticus is a SE syndrome

TABLE 1: **Etiologies for status epilepticus**

Variant of status epilepticus	Etiology
Acute symptomatic SE	Infective meningoencephalitis; trauma; anoxia; acute stroke (including hemorrhage and cortical venous sinus thrombosis); vasculitis; autoimmune encephalitis (paraneoplastic and nonparaneoplastic autoantibody mediated); central nervous system tumors including metastases; neurocysticercosis granulomas; metabolic (hyponatremia, hypocalcemia, hypoglycemia, nonketotic hyperosmolar state); substance abuse/withdrawal (alcohol, cocaine); proconvulsant medications (cephalosporins, e.g., cefepime, quinolones, tricyclic antidepressants, lithium); neurometabolic disorders (Reye's syndrome, mitochondrial cytopathy)
Remote symptomatic SE	Cerebral gliotic scars (secondary to perinatal insults, remote-strokes, trauma, healed granulomas, brain tumor surgery, radiotherapy); post-inflammatory (Rasmussen's encephalitis); progressive etiologies (e.g. progressive myoclonus epilepsy, storage disorders)
Idiopathic/cryptogenic SE	Unknown etiology (e.g., febrile status epilepticus; new onset refractory status epilepticus)
SE in established epilepsy (low drug levels, *de novo*)	Idiopathic epilepsies (juvenile absence/myoclonic epilepsies) Symptomatic epilepsies (malformations of cortical development, chromosomal aberrations) Epileptic encephalopathy (Lennox-Gastaut syndrome)

SE, status epilepticus.

described in adult patients who present with severe secondary generalized seizures amounting to SE and is of an uncertain etiology.[34] This and similar forms described in school-going children and adolescents forms of RSE that come under the rubric of fever-induced refractory epileptic encephalopathy syndrome (FIRES) are known to be extremely refractory to standard management protocols and have high morbidity and mortality.[35] The etiology for these conditions is speculative at best and believed to have genetic or immunological bases.

TREATMENT

The principles of management of SE are centered on a rapid identification and correction of inciting yet reversible or treatable causes, maintenance of cerebral and systemic homeostasis targeting early cessation of SE.

Prehospital Management

The studies, which have looked into the prehospital management of SE, have demonstrated the safety and efficacy of rectal diazepam (15–20 mg as rectal gel) in adults. Other drugs which form part of the armamentarium include IV lorazepam (4 mg), diazepam (5 mg), and buccal/intramuscular (IM) midazolam (10 mg), all of which have demonstrated good safety profiles when utilized in the prehospital setting by paramedics. Efficacy on application via the IM route is also established.[36] Ideally, paramedical expertise is warranted even in this setting.

Emergent Care

Maintenance of airway, breathing, and circulation is of paramount importance in patients presenting with SE, considering the consequent neuronal injury that may prove to be irreversible. One should bear in mind emergent etiologies that include hypoglycemia, hyponatremia, hypocalcemia, hypomagnesemia, acidosis, hyperthermia, and last but not the least, a common pathway leading to hypoxic neuronal damage. In a situation of suspected alcohol abuse, IV thiamine 100 mg bolus along with dextrose solution should be administered. As hypoxia may not be clinically apparent, supplementary oxygen is recommended in all patients as a precautionary measure. Emergent tests ought to include blood gases, electrocardiogram, glucose, renal and hepatic functions, calcium, magnesium, creatine phosphokinase, complete blood count, clotting screen, and AED concentrations. In suspected acute meningoencephalitis, a cerebrospinal fluid analysis with specific tests for bacterial, viral, or parasitic etiologies should be contemplated. Cerebral decongestants should be considered in the presence of clinical or imaging evidence of intracranial hypertension. Vascular etiologies, such as stroke, venous infarction, or intracerebral hemorrhage, require targeted therapy. When SE and consequent coma is of uncertain etiology, serum should be stored for toxicology or virology or other future analyses.

Anti-epileptic Drug Therapy in Status Epilepticus

Most intensive care unit (ICU)/hospital treatment protocols in SE are focused on a staged approach.[37,38] The first- and second-line drugs included in this stage-based management are largely judged on their rapid and predictable pharmacokinetic profile, efficacy, and cardiorespiratory safety. The detailed protocol of therapy and the dosages are provided in flowchart 1 and table 2. The basic principles for inhospital management of SE include:

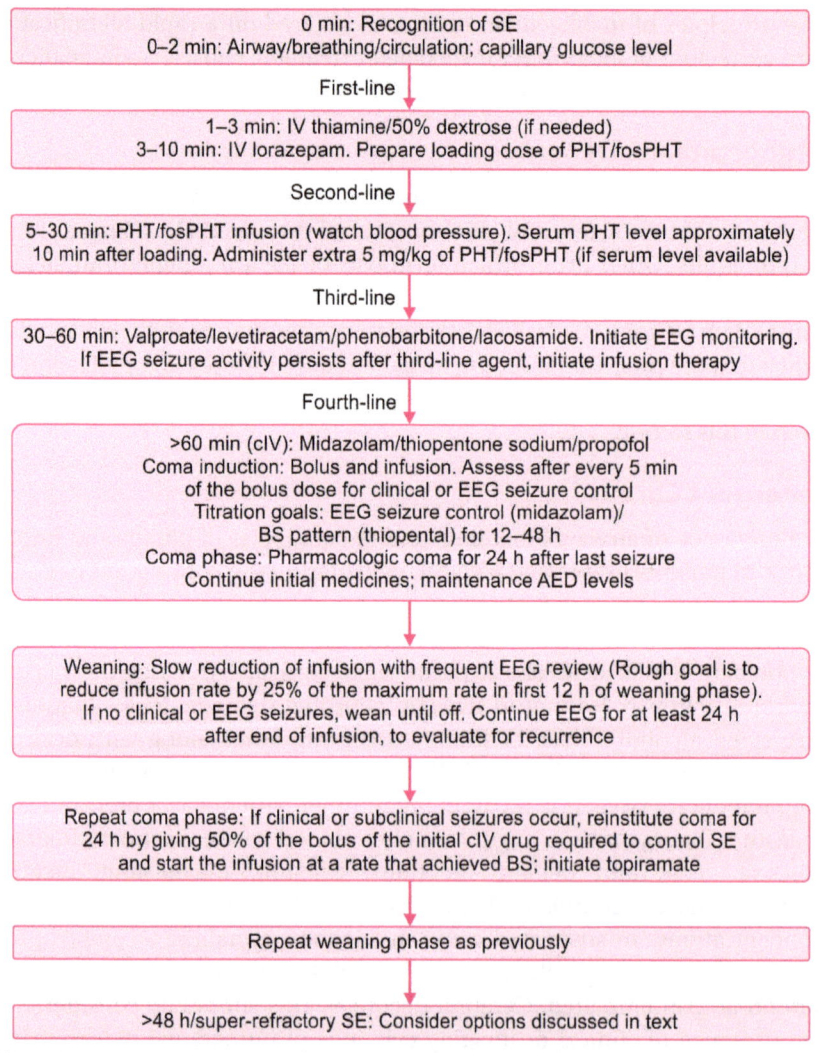

cIV, continuous intravenous infusion; SE, status epilepticus; EEG, electroencephalography; AED, anti-epileptic drugs; PHT, phenytoin; fosPHT, fosphenytoin; BS, burst-suppression.

FLOWCHART 1: A pragmatic algorithm in status epilepticus

TABLE 2: Anti-epileptic drugs used in the treatment of status epilepticus and their doses

Anti-epileptic drug	Dose
First-line (IV)	
• Lorazepam	• 0.1 mg/kg bolus @2 mg/min
• Diazepam	• 0.2 mg/kg bolus @4 mg/min
• Midazolam	• 0.05–0.2 mg/kg @2 mg/min
Second-line (IV)	
Phenytoin	• 15–20 mg/kg @50 mg/min
	• Maintenance = 4–7 mg/kg/day (IV/PO)
Fosphenytoin	• 15–20 mg/kg PE @75–150 mg/min
	• Target phenytoin level = 15–20 µg/mL
Third-line (IV)	
Levetiracetam	• 20–30 mg/kg bolus over 15 min, followed by maintenance dosing 1,500 mg BID (IV/PO)
Sodium valproate	• 15–30 mg/kg bolus @up to 6 mg/kg/min, followed by maintenance dosing 500 mg TID (IV/PO)
	• Target valproate level = 50–100 µg/mL
Phenobarbitone (ventilator on standby)	• 20 mg/kg bolus @75 mg/min, followed by initial maintenance dosing 60 mg TID (IV/PO)
	• Target phenobarbitone level = 20–40 µg/mL
Lacosamide	• 200 mg @50 mg/min; 200 mg BID (IV/PO)
Fourth-line (cIV)	
Midazolam (optional third-line treatment if ventilator on standby)	• Loading: 0.1–0.2 mg/kg (maximum, 10 mg at a time) repeat bolus—if clinical seizures persist 5 min after initial bolus, then administer additional bolus of 0.2 mg/kg bolus and continue infusion. Repeat bolus every 5 min till total midazolam bolus dose reaches 2 mg/kg
	• Maintenance cIV dose: 0.05–0.4 mg/kg/h
	• Maximum cIV dose: increase infusion rate (with each bolus) of midazolam by 0.05–0.1 mg/kg/h to a maximum infusion rate of up to 3 mg/kg/h
Thiopental sodium	• Loading: 3–5 mg/kg at 0.2–0.4 mg/kg/min
	• Maintenance cIV dose: 3.0–5.0 mg/kg/h
	• Maximum cIV dose: 5.0 mg/kg/h
Propofol	• Loading: 1–2 mg/kg at 10 mg/min
	• Maintenance cIV dose: 2–10 mg/kg/h
	• Maximum cIV dose: 15 mg/kg/h
Topiramate (PO)	• 10 mg/kg NG loading dose followed by 5 mg/kg NG divided BID
	• Dose range: 300–1,600 mg

IV, intravenous route of administration; cIV, continuous intravenous infusion; BID, twice daily; TID, thrice daily; PE, phenytoin equivalent dose (1.5 times of phenytoin dose); PO, peroral route; NG, nasogastric route of administration

- Rapid treatment of clinical and electrographic seizures with treatment of underlying etiology
- Lorazepam IV, midazolam IM, and rectal diazepam are the first-line drugs
- The second-line drugs may include IV fosphenytoin, sodium valproate, lacosamide, or levetiracetam or if in ICU, phenobarbitone
- Anesthetic drugs should be titrated to burst suppression or isoelectric EEG
- Duration of treatment should be at least 24–48 hours before weaning anesthetic drugs and maintenance drugs should be provided
- Transfer to a neurocritical care unit experienced in long-term management of seizures as well as systemic complications of management.

First-line Drugs

Heterogeneous management protocols are implemented across centers due to a paucity of randomized controlled trials comparing various first-line medications in SE. In most protocols, IV benzodiazepines are of first choice.[37] Lorazepam or diazepam have shown equivalent benefits in studies with the former evidenced to have a better safety profile. Intravenous midazolam has gained widespread acceptance and comparison trials are emerging.[39] As mentioned previously, a recent study demonstrated efficacy of IM midazolam in prehospital seizure cessation in comparison to IV lorazepam.[36] An important consideration is the issue of respiratory or cardiovascular decompensation that is an inherent risk with benzodiazepines or even phenytoin, especially in children and the elderly due to which close monitoring is mandatory. Evidence has emerged including an open-labeled randomized study from India that has established efficacy and safety of levetiracetam in comparison to lorazepam in children and adults.[40,41] In the context of a hemodynamically unstable patient, levetiracetam could prove to be an acceptable alternative as a first-line agent during an impending or established SE.

Second-line Drugs

The IV agents available are phenytoin, valproate, levetiracetam, and lacosamide.[37,42] Intravenous fosphenytoin or phenytoin is generally preferred world-over as first choice, if the seizures are not controlled with benzodiazepines. Fosphenytoin is preferred over phenytoin due to the favorable side effect profile, especially lack of thrombophlebitis and relative hemodynamic safety. Insufficient data is available on the comparative efficacy of phenytoin and fosphenytoin. A head-to-head comparison between phenytoin, valproate, and levetiracetam revealed noninferiority of phenytoin and levetiracetam was found have inferior efficacy over valproate to control SE.[43] Efficacy of lacosamide is based on observational and retrospective series.[42,44] A couple of randomized controlled studies from India concluded almost similar efficacy between phenytoin and valproic acid although there are no studies comparing levetiracetam or lacosamide with these agents.[45,46] Oral topiramate has been compared to phenytoin in one randomized trial and has been found to have equivalent efficacy in adults.[47] In the absence of conclusive evidence, pragmatic selection of one or two of these agents, preferably with IV formulations is warranted based on the clinical situation and these need to be administered orally once SE is controlled. Seizure clusters with impending SE may be controlled by coadministration of an alternative second-line agent, thereby avoiding the requirement of third-line therapy.

Third-line Medications in Refractory Status Epilepticus

At this stage, continuous IV infusion (cIV) of general anesthetic medications need to be considered after establishing airway protection via intubation and elective ventilation.[37,39] While a majority of SE are well-controlled upon initiating this intervention, failure to do so may be a consequence of systemic side effects or failure to achieve the defined targeted dosage. Upon withdrawal of these agents, recurrence of seizures or SE may be seen in 0.3–9% cases.[37] Anesthetic agents used in RSE include midazolam, thiopental sodium/pentobarbital, and propofol.[37,48] Most critical care units prefer midazolam in view of the ease of administration, control of seizures, lesser rate of withdrawal seizures, and fewer side effects are exhibited by this drug as compared to the other two due to the lack of significant fat storage.[48] There is insufficient evidence to recommend one anesthetic agent over another in terms of its efficacy or tendency for relapse. Attempts at weaning/cessation of anesthetic agents are made once electrographic status has been controlled for 24–48 hours and therapeutic levels of at least two conventional AED have been achieved. A cycle of weaning and then reinstituting anesthesia, if seizures recur, may happen every 24–48 hours. This is highlighted in the EEG series depicted in figure 1. If seizures recur, it may be necessary to treat longer and taper more slowly the next time while maintaining high therapeutic levels of other AED, however, this decision is less often protocol driven and more individualized. There are no large multicentric studies or controlled trials regarding the practice or duration of recycling anesthetic agents. Propofol is associated with potentially fatal "propofol infusion syndrome" of rhabdomyolysis, hepatitis, and metabolic acidosis. This is consequent to its depression of cellular and mitochondrial homeostasis as a result of which children and patients comedicated with catecholamines and steroids need to be carefully monitored for this dreaded condition. The target of anesthetic treatment in SE is to achieve burst-suppression pattern in the EEG although there exists an argument for targeting only background suppression along with control of clinical seizures. Electroencephalography is pertinent at this level due to the high

Epilepsy

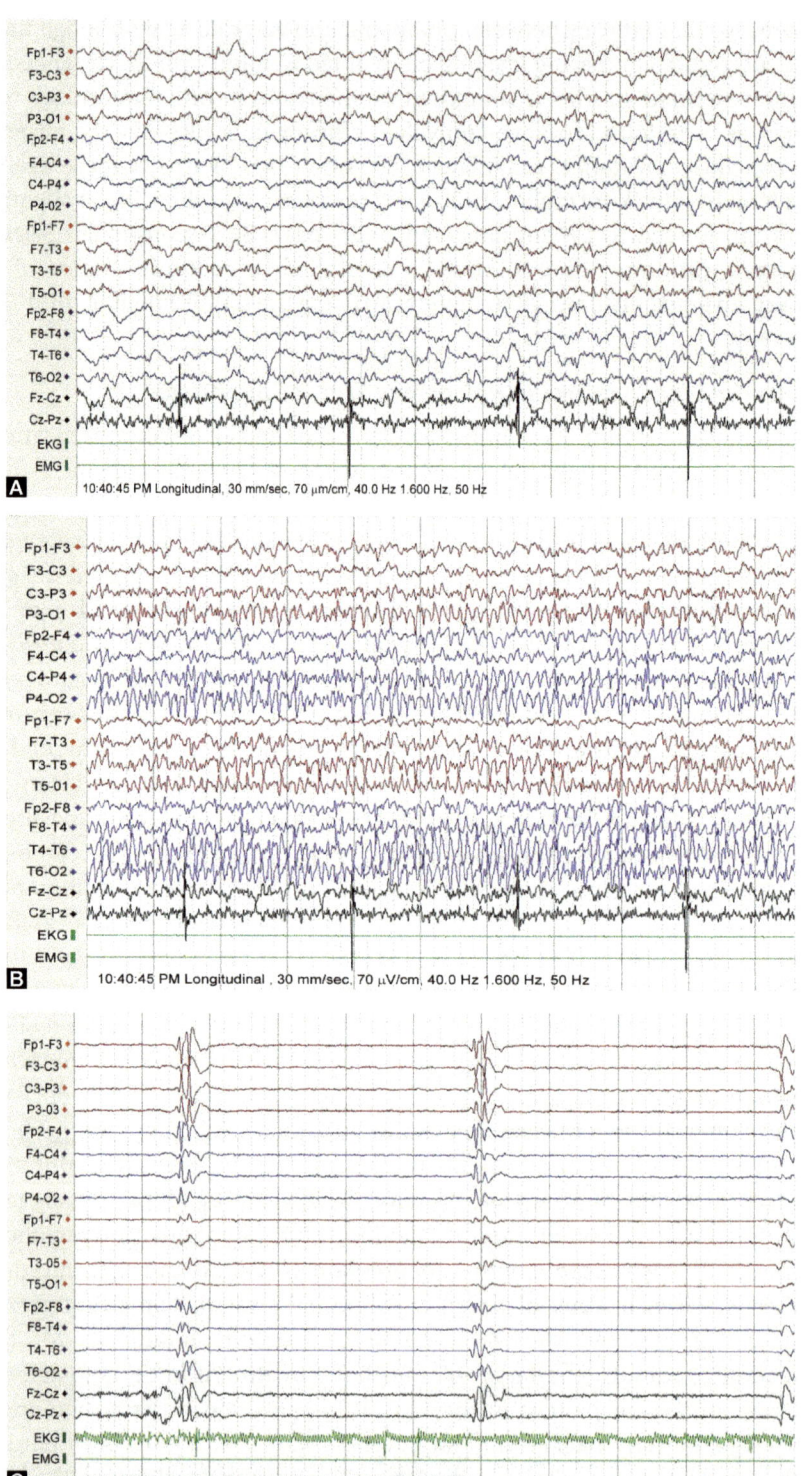

Continued

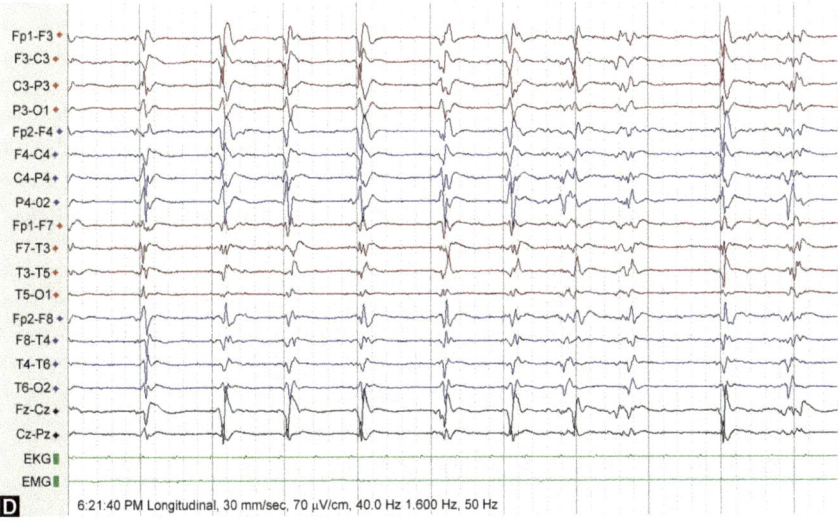

FIG. 1: Serial electroencephalography (EEGs) in a 28-year-old lady who developed super-refractory status epilepticus following viral encephalitis: **A**, EEG showing bilateral independent periodic lateralized epileptiform discharges; **B**, evolution of electrographic seizures associated with deep coma (nonconvulsive status epilepticus) on intravenous midazolam; **C**, pharmacological burst suppression using intravenous thiopentone infusion; **D**, generalized periodic epileptiform discharges upon withdrawal of thiopentone with persistence of coma. The patient was treated with recycling of intravenous anesthetic agents (midazolam, thiopentone, ketamine) in addition to five anti-epileptic drugs. Additionally, corticosteroids and intravenous immunoglobulin was also administered. Patient recovered to normal occupational functioning after 43 days of super-refractory status epilepticus

incidence of "electromechanical dissociation" wherein the patient may continue to be in deep coma with persistence of electrographic seizure activity and absence of subtle or florid-convulsive manifestations may be noted. A meta-analysis of 193 patients with RSE found that as opposed to seizure suppression, background suppression was significantly associated with fewer recurrences, but at the expense of a higher incidence of hypotension and systemic side effects and without a benefit on mortality.[39] A single-center retrospective study of 47 patients with RSE also found outcome to be independent of the extent of EEG suppression.[20] Another study found that suppression of seizures, as opposed to burst or complete suppression, was associated with better functional outcome.[49]

Systemic complications a physician should monitor during the course of management of RSE are summarized in table 3.

TABLE 3: Systemic complications of ongoing seizures and management of status epilepticus

Pulmonary	Hypoxia, pulmonary edema, acute respiratory distress syndrome, collapse, pneumothorax, tracheostomy related
Cardiovascular	Brady-/tachyarrhythmias, hypotension, systolic dysfunction
Hematological	Deep vein thrombosis, pulmonary embolism, leukopenia, thrombocytopenia, anemia
Renal	Acid-base and electrolyte imbalance, renal failure (acute tubular necrosis), rhabdomyolysis
Infections	Ventilator-associated pneumonia, sepsis, pseudomembranous colitis, urinary tract infection
Gastrointestinal	Paralytic ileus, drug-induced hepatitis, hypoalbuminemia
Musculoskeletal	Critical illness neuromyopathy
Endocrinological	Stress hyperglycemia, diabetes insipidus
Dermatological	Decubitus ulcers, Stevens-Johnson syndrome, drug rash

Super-refractory Status Epilepticus

Super-refractory SE is an operationally new terminology used to define SE that continues for 24 hours or more after the initiation of anesthesia, including those cases in which the SE recurs on the reduction or withdrawal of anesthesia.[50] Options are mostly based on anecdotal reports and observational case series. In a small series on super-refractory SE, ketamine was demonstrated to successfully abate SE in 82% based on its antagonistic action on NMDA receptors. The agent is also believed to have a neuroprotective role although this postulate requires further study.[51] Anecdotal case reports also support the use of inhalational anesthetics such as isoflurane and desflurane and agents such as IV magnesium, oral pyridoxine.[50,52] Immunomodulatory regimens-utilizing steroids, IV immunoglobulin, and plasma exchange are effective in occult or antibody positive autoimmune SE.[53] Ketogenic diet may be efficacious in SE due to epileptic encephalopathy and in FIRES. Hypothermia targeted to cooling of core temperature to 32–35°C, preferably delivered by endovascular means, may potentiate neuroprotection, if administered early, but one should be aware of the various systemic complications.[50] Epilepsy surgery has been used in many centers for RSE and its rationale is focused on identification of surgically remediable syndromes using high-resolution magnetic resonance imaging. This may identify epileptogenic substrates that can be safely resected or disconnected such as malformations of cortical development or focal encephalitis such as Rasmussen's encephalitis (Fig. 2). Magnetic and electrical stimulation therapies, like transcranial magnetic stimulation, vagus nerve stimulation, deep brain stimulation, and electroconvulsive therapy, are experimental forms of treatment used in SE with only anecdotal evidence.[50]

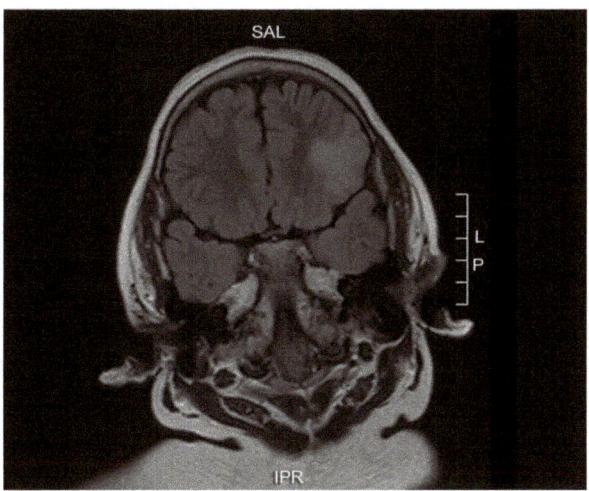

FIG. 2: Fluid-attenuated inversion recovery coronal magnetic resonance imaging (MRI) of a 9-year-old boy who presented with clustering of complex partial seizures of left hemispheric origin and evolved into complex partial status epilepticus. Image shows gyral and white matter edema over the left inferior frontal gyrus and frontal operculum. In view of recurrent episodes of complex partial status epilepticus not responding to multiple anti-epileptic drug, steroids, immunoglobulin, and intravenous midazolam, the patients was taken up for an emergent motor cortex sparing functional left hemispherotomy (anterior quadrantic disconnection). Postoperatively, he continues to have minor right upper limb simple partial seizures with preserved motor and language functions and has resumed schooling. Histopathology confirmed the MRI suspicion of Rasmussen's encephalitis

OUTCOME

Mortality from SE in various studies is up to 20%.[1,5,37] Major determinant of the outcome in SE is the underlying etiology. In one study, which specifically looked into the duration elapsed before instituting correct treatment in SE, a duration of less than 10 hours was associated with a better overall outcome, but this was not significant once etiology, presentation in a comatose state and type of SE were accounted for.[54] In a study on convulsive SE from India demonstrated the overall mortality at 10.5%.[33] Also, longer duration of seizures was associated with increased morbidity. These facts reflect on the importance of emergent treatment of SE at the primary healthcare contact point. A prognostic scale referred to as the Status Epilepticus Severity Score (STESS) offers an objective perspective in terms of increasing age, depth of coma, absence of prior history of seizures and presentation as NCSE to be adverse indicators although this requires further validation in multicentric studies.[55]

A study of SE in 84 patients from our Institute over a period of 10 years has provided us valuable insights.[56] In this retrospective study, single episode of SE was treated in 72 patients (86%) and multiple SE events, ranging from

2-6 events/patient were managed in 12 patients (14%). Mean age of the cohort was 24.1 ± 20.3 years and 63% were males. The subtypes included convulsive SE in 98 (90.7%), NCSE in 7 (6.5%), and myoclonic status in 3 (2.8%). Around 60% events were of remote symptomatic etiology, 16% were acute symptomatic, 16% were of unexplained etiology, and 8% were progressive symptomatic. In 85 events (79%), SE could be aborted with first- and second-line drugs. The remaining 23 events (21%) progressed to RSE, among which 13 (56%) were controlled with cIV midazolam infusion. Case fatality rate in our study was 11%; more than one-fifth of patients developed neurological sequelae and 67% recovered to baseline functional status. Acute symptomatic SE, older age, altered sensorium at the time of admission, and delayed hospitalization were predictors of poor outcome.

CONCLUSION

It is thus of paramount importance to recognize SE in both its convulsive and nonconvulsive or subtle forms. Decision-making as well as prompt initiation of first- and second-line therapy is critical to achieve desirable outcomes and early referral is important when ventilatory care and IV anesthesia are anticipated. Emergent EEG is an accepted standard-of-care, not only in the recognition of nonconvulsive SE but also when IV anesthesia is to be initiated with midazolam or barbiturates. Identification and amelioration of the initial precipitating insult is likely to impact the outcome of SE, especially in acute symptomatic SE. State funding is mandatory to equip basic facilities at primary healthcare centers, so as to avoid inordinate delays in the initial management of SE. Status epilepticus may become intractable until the underlying etiology is identified and treated thereby emphasizing the importance of early referral to a neurocritical care unit. Medical complications are common and they may worsen outcome. Nevertheless, when SE, especially its refractory and super-refractory forms can be aborted, functional recovery may occur over time, even after weeks or months of SE. Thus, prolonged aggressive treatment is generally justified. There is a need for multicentric collaborative studies to judge what constitutes an adequate IV anesthesia protocol as well as newer interventional strategies focused on neuroprotective and anti-"epileptogenic" strategies in the refractory forms of SE. Reducing the morbidity and mortality due to SE remains a challenge for the future.

REFERENCES

1. DeLorenzo RJ, Hauser WA, Towne AR. A prospective, population based epidemiologic study of status epilepticus in Richmond, Virginia. Neurology. 1996;46:1029-35.
2. Hesdorffer DC, Logroscino G, Cascino G, Annegers JF, Hauser WA. Incidence of status epilepticus in Rochester, Minnesota, 1965-1984. Neurology. 1998;50:735-41.
3. C oeytaux A, Jallon P, Galobardes B, Morabia A. Incidence of status epilepticus in French-speaking Switzerland: EPISTAR. Neurology. 2000;55:693-7.

4. Knake S, Rosenow F, Vescovi M, Oertel WH, Mueller HH, WirbatzA, et al. Incidence of status epilepticus in adults in Germany: a prospective, population-based study. Epilepsia. 2001;40:759-62.
5. Vignatelli L, Tonon C, D'Alessandro R. Bologna Group for the Study of Status Epilepticus. Incidence and short-term prognosis of status epilepticus in adults in Bologna, Italy. Epilepsia. 2003;44:964-8.
6. Neligan A, Shorvon S. Frequency and prognosis of convulsive status epilepticus of different causes: A systematic review. Arch Neurol. 2010;67:931-40.
7. Chin RF, Neville BG, Peckham C, Bedford H, Wade A, Scott RC. Incidence, cause, and short-term outcome of convulsive status epilepticus in childhood: prospective population-based study. Lancet. 2006;368:222-9.
8. Commission on Classification and Terminology of the International League Against Epilepsy. Proposal for revised clinical and electroencephalographic classification of epileptic seizures. Epilepsia. 1981;22:489-501.
9. Berg AT, Berkovic SF, Brodie MJ, Buchhalter J, Cross JH, van Emde Boas W, et al. Revised terminology and concepts for organization of seizures and epilepsies: report of the ILAE Commission on Classification and Terminology, 2005–2009. Epilepsia. 2010;51:676-85.
10. Trinka E, Höfler J, Zerbs A. Causes of status epilepticus. Epilepsia. 2012;53:127-38.
11. Lowenstein DH, Bleck T, Macdonald RL. It's time to revise the definition of status epilepticus. Epilepsia. 1999;40:120-2.
12. Mazarati AM, Wasterlain CG, Sankar R, Shin D. Self-sustaining status epilepticus after brief electrical stimulation of the perforant path. Brain Res. 1998;801:251-3.
13. Bauer G, Trinka E. Nonconvulsive status epilepticus and coma. Epilepsia. 2010;51:177-90.
14. Shorvon S. The management of status epilepticus. J Neurol Neurosurg Psychiatry. 2001;70:22-7.
15. Chen J, Wasterlain C. Status epilepticus: pathophysiology and management in adults. Lancet Neurol. 2006;5:246-56.
16. Theodore WH, Porter RJ, Albert P, Kelley K, Bromfield E, Devinsky O, et al. The secondarily generalized tonic-clonic seizure: a videotape analysis. Neurology. 1994;44:1403-7.
17. Delorenzo RJ, Garnett LK, Towne AR, DeLorenzo RJ, Garnett LK, Towne AR, et al. Comparison of status epilepticus with prolonged seizure episodes lasting from 10 to 29 minutes. Epilepsia. 1999;40:164-9.
18. Wasterlain CG, Mazarati AM, Naylor D, Niquet J, Liu H, Suchomelova L, et al. Short-term plasticity of hippocampal neuropeptides and neuronal circuitry in experimental status epilepticus. Epilepsia. 2002;43:20-9.
19. Holtkamp M, Othman J, Buchheim K, Meierkord H. Predictors and prognosis of refractory status epilepticus treated in a neurological intensive care unit. J Neurol Neurosurg Psychiatry. 2005;76:534-9.
20. Rossetti AO, Logroscino G, Bromfield EB. Refractory status epilepticus: effect of treatment aggressiveness on prognosis. Arch Neurol. 2005;62:1698-702.
21. Treiman DM, Walton NY, Kendrick C. A progressive sequence of electro-encephalographic changes during generalized convulsive status epilepticus. Epilepsy Res. 1990;5:49-60.
22. Mazarati AM, Wasterlain CG. N-methyl-D-asparate receptor antagonists abolish the maintenance phase of self-sustaining status epilepticus in rat. Neurosci Lett. 1999;265:187-90.
23. Kapur J, Macdonald RL. Rapid seizure-induced reduction of benzodiazepine and Zn2+ sensitivity of hippocampal dentate granule cell GABAA receptors. J Neurosci. 1997;17:7532-40.

24. Naylor DE, Liu H, Wasterlain CG. Trafficking of GABA(A) receptors, loss of inhibition, and a mechanism for pharmacoresistance in status epilepticus. J Neurosci. 2005;25:7724-33.
25. Hamil NE, Cock HR, Walker MC. Acute down-regulation of adenosine A(1) receptor activity in status epilepticus. Epilepsia. 2012;53:177-88.
26. Aminoff MJ, Simon RP. Status epilepticus: causes, clinical features and consequences in 98 patients. Am J Med. 1980;69:659-66.
27. Lowenstein DH, Alldredge BH. Status epilepticus at an urban public hospital in the 1980s. Neurology. 1993;143:483-8.
28. De Lorenzo RJ, Pellock JM, Towne AR, Bogges JG. Epidemiology of status epilepticus. J Clin Neurophysiol. 1995;12:316-25.
29. Fountain NB. Status epilepticus: risk factors and complications. Epilepsia. 2000;41:S23-30.
30. Vignatelli L, Tonon C, D'Alessandro R. Bologna Group for the Study of Status Epilepticus. Incidence and short-term prognosis of status epilepticus in adults in Bologna, Italy. Epilepsia. 2003;44:964-8.
31. Mhodj I, Nadiaye M, Sene F, Sow PS, Sow HD, Diagana M, et al. Treatment of status epilepticus in a developing country. Neurophysiol Clin. 2000;30:165-9.
32. Garzon E, Fernandes RM, Sakamoto AC. Analysis of clinical characteristic and risk factors for mortality in human status epilepticus. Seizure. 2003;12:237-45.
33. Murthy JMK, Jayalaxmi S, Kanikannan M. Convulsive status epilepticus: clinical profile in a developing country. Epilepsia. 2007;48:2217-23.
34. Costello DJ, Kilbride RD, Cole AJ. Cryptogenic new onset refractory status epilepticus (NORSE) in adults—Infectious or not? J Neurol Sci. 2009;277:26-31.
35. Ismail FY, Kossoff EH. AERRPS, DESC, NORSE, FIRES: multi-labeling or distinct epileptic entities? Epilepsia. 2011;52:e185-9.
36. Silbergleit R, Durkalski V, Lowenstein D, Conwit R, Pancioli A, Palesch Y, et al. Intramuscular versus intravenous therapy for prehospital status epilepticus. N Engl J Med. 2012;366:591-600.
37. Shorvon S, Baulac M, Cross H, Trinka E, Walker M. The drug treatment of status epilepticus in Europe: consensus document from a workshop at the first London Colloquium on Status Epilepticus. Epilepsia. 2008;49:1277-85.
38. Cock HR, ESETT Group. Established status epilepticus treatment trial (ESETT). Epilepsia. 2011;52:50-2.
39. Claassen J. Treatment of refractory status epilepticus with pentobarbital, propofol, or midazolam: a systematic review. Epilepsia. 2002;43:146-53.
40. Misra UK, Kalita J, Maurya PK. Levetiracetam versus lorazepam in status epilepticus: a randomized, open labeled pilot study. J Neurol. 2012;259:645-8.
41. Mctague A, Kneen R, Kumar R, Spinty S, Appleton R. Intravenous levetiracetam in acute repetitive seizures and status epilepticus in children: Experience from a children's hospital. Seizure. 2012;21:529-34.
42. Hçfler J, Unterberger I, Dobesberger J, Kuchukhidze G, Walser G, Trinka E. Intravenous lacosamide in status epilepticus and seizure clusters. Epilepsia. 2011;52:148-52.
43. Alvarz V, Januel J-M, Burnand B, Rossetti AO. Second line status epilepticus treatment: comparison of phenytoin, valproate and levetiracetam. Epilepsia. 2011;52:1292-6.
44. Trinka E. What is the evidence to use new intravenous AEDs in status epilepticus? Epilepsia. 2011;52:35-8.
45. Misra UK, Kalitha J, Rajesh P. Sodium valproate versus phenytoin in status epilepticus: a pilot study. Neurology. 2006;67:340-2.
46. Agarwal P, Kumar N, Chandra R, Gupta G, Antony A, Garg N. Randomised study of intravenous valproate and phenytoin in status epilepticus. Seizure. 2007;16:527-32.

47. Synowiec AS, Yandora KA, Yenugadhati V. The efficacy of topiramate in adult refractory status epilepticus: experience of a tertiary care center. Epilepsy Res. 2012;98:232-7.
48. Shorvon S, Trinka E. Status epilepticus—making progress. Epilepsia. 2011;52:1-2.
49. Hocker S, Britton JW, Mandrekar J, Wijdicks EF, Rabinstein AA. Predictors of outcome in refractory status epilepticus. Arch Neurol. 2012;8:1-6.
50. Shorvon S, Ferlisi M. The treatment of super-refractory status epilepticus: a critical review of available therapies and a clinical treatment protocol. Brain. 2011;134:2802-18.
51. Höfler J, Rohracher A, Kalss G, Zimmermann G, Dobesberger J, Pilz G, et al. (S)-ketamine in refractory and super-refractory status epilepticus: A retrospective study. CNS Drugs. 2016;30:869-76.
52. Zeiler FA, Zeiler KJ, Teitelbaum J, Gillman LM, West M. Modern inhalational anesthetics for refractory status epilepticus. Can J Neurol Sci. 2015;42:106-15.
53. LoPinto-Khoury C, Sperling M. Autoimmune status epilepticus. Curr Treat Opt Neurol. 2013;15:545-56.
54. Drislane F, Blum A, Lopez M, Gautam S, Schomer D. Duration of refractory status epilepticus and outcome: Loss of prognostic utility after several hours. Epilepsia. 2009;50:1566-71.
55. Rossetti AO, Logroscino G, Milligan TA, Michaelides C, Ruffieux C, Bromfield EB. Status Epilepticus Severity Score (STESS): a tool to orient early treatment strategy. J Neurol. 2008;255:1561-6.
56. Hassan H, Rajiv KR, Menon R, Menon D, Nair M, Radhakrishnan A. An audit of the predictors of outcome in status epilepticus from a resource-poor country: a comparison with developed countries. Epileptic Disord. 2016;18:163-72.

CHAPTER 10

Epilepsy Surgery

Biji Bahuleyan

INTRODUCTION

Surgical treatment of epilepsy has transformed tremendously in the recent past with advancement in technology and development of newer surgical techniques. A neurosurgeon performing epilepsy surgery should have appropriate training in this field. The functional and microsurgical anatomy of human brain varies considerably. The success of epilepsy surgery is to perform the procedure with good seizure outcome without neurological deficits.

Epilepsy surgery is indicated for patients with medically refractory epilepsy who are evaluated and selected for the procedure by a "comprehensive epilepsy team". Even though the definition of refractory epilepsy can vary depending on the socioeconomic status of the patient, a rough rule would be a patient with two or more disabling seizures per month for a period of 2 years and has failed trials of two anti-epileptic monotherapy and one poly therapy during this period. About 20% of patients diagnosed with seizures are refractory to medications and majority of them ultimately become surgical candidates.[1] Epilepsy surgery aims at manipulating the abnormal part of the brain that generates seizures with an aim to stop or reduce seizures, ultimately improving their quality of life.

Refractory epilepsy should be evaluated and managed only by a team of healthcare providers that constitute a "comprehensive epilepsy team". This is important because management of these patients is complex and is much more than treating epilepsy alone. The team should include an epileptologist, neurosurgeon, neuroradiologist, psychiatrist, psychologist, and a social worker.

The presurgical evaluation of drug-resistant epilepsy includes both noninvasive and invasive modalities. The objective of these tests is to establish a clinical, radiological, and electrophysiological concordance with respect to patient's seizure semiology. The success of epilepsy surgery is based on the ability of the treating team to establish this concordance and when present, is associated with excellent seizure outcome. The noninvasive tests include computerized tomography (CT) scans, magnetic resonance imaging (MRI) scans, video electroencephalogram (EEG) monitoring, single photon emission computed tomography, positron emission tomography scans, and Wada test. Magnetic resonance imaging is considered the first imaging modality of choice for these patients as this can identify structural lesions.[2] Magnetic resonance imaging scans should be performed preferably in a center with a stronger magnet to improve the resolution of the images to pick up lesions and should be read by a neuroradiologist. The invasive modalities of investigations include placement of invasive electrodes either on the surface (surface electrodes) or deeper (depth electrodes) areas of the brain by an open surgical procedure. Stereo EEG is an old invasive modality that fell out of favor in the past; however, is gaining popularity in the recent years. Stereo EEG is considered in patients with intractable seizures where the lesion cannot be identified on an MRI. In stereo EEG, multiple electrodes are placed stereotactically or with the help of a neurorobot into deeper regions of the brain that is hypothesized to have the seizure onset.

From a pathological stand point of view, the commonest cause of refractory epilepsy is mesial temporal sclerosis (MTS). Other lesions include malformations of cortical development (focal cortical dysplasia, microgyria, pachygyria, agyria, schizencephaly, hemimegalencephaly), hamartomas, infections (tuberculosis, neurocysticercosis), inflammatory lesions (Rasmussen's encephalitis), traumatic lesions, vascular malformations (Sturge Weber syndrome, cavernoma), and neoplastic lesions. The neoplastic lesions causing drug-resistant seizures are dysembryoplastic neuroepithelial tumor, ganglioglioma, and glioma.

Broadly, epilepsy surgery is categorized into two—resections and disconnections. Generally, resections are performed in noneloquent regions of the brain for focal seizures. Examples of resections are amygdalohippocampectomy and anterior temporal lobectomy. Resections are also done for lesions (mentioned above) that cause seizures. On the other hand, disconnections are done when eloquent brain is involved in the origin or propagation of seizures or when the seizure onset is multifocal. The disconnective procedures disconnect the white matter tracts that propagate seizures. Disconnection thus helps inhibiting the spread of impulses from one region of the hemisphere to the other or between two hemispheres. Examples of disconnective procedures are corpus callosotomy, hemispherotomy, and multiple subpial transections.

At surgery, various special recordings are used to enable the surgeon and the neurologist to guide and to assess the completeness of resection. The neurophysiological recordings used during surgery are the electrocorticography (ECoG), cortical stimulation for locating specific regions of the brain (sensory-motor cortex, speech area), somatosensory evoked potential, etc. Some centers use intraoperative MRI scans to assess the completeness of resection of lesions.

TEMPORAL LOBE EPILEPSY SURGERY

Temporal lobe epilepsy is broadly classified into two—the neocortical (lateral temporal) and mesial temporal lobe epilepsy. These two epileptic syndromes have some common characteristics; however, there are definite features that help epileptologists distinguish them. The mesial temporal lobe epilepsy presents with aura, staring, automatisms, and posturing, where as the neocortical seizures present with auditory hallucinations and in the dominant hemisphere, post ictal aphasia. The clinical and EEG features of these two syndromes are different, and hence, localization is often not very difficult.

The commonest cause of epilepsy and temporal lobe epilepsy per se is the MTS (Fig. 1). Mesial temporal sclerosis is characterized by anomalies in the amygdala, hippocampus, fornix, mammilary bodies, thalamus and neocortex, and the entire hemisphere. Rarely, temporal lobe epilepsy can be secondary to other lesions in the temporal lobe that are listed earlier in this chapter.

Microsurgically, the mesial temporal lobe includes the amygdala, hippocampus, and parahippocampus and the neocortex involves the rest of the temporal lobe. The resections for temporal lobe epilepsy can be either removal of the mesial temporal lobe, neocortex, or both. The standard temporal lobectomy, first proposed by Falconer[3] involved removal of the mesial temporal lobe and the neocortex. However, in patients with a clear unilateral

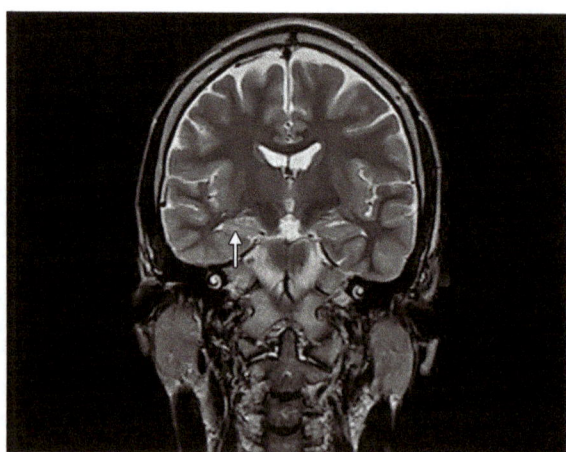

FIG. 1: Coronal MRI scan of the brain showing atrophy of the right hippocampus with intrinsic signal intensity changes. Note the atrophy of the ipsilateral hemisphere including the temporal lobe

mesial temporal seizure onset, selective resection of the mesial temporal lobe, the "selective amygdalohippocampectomy (SAH)" is a valid surgical option. Niemeyer described the technique of SAH, retaining the neocortex.[4] Later numerous modifications of SAH were proposed depending on the anatomical route through which the mesial temporal lobe is approached. From the literature available today addressing the seizure outcome, it is difficult to ascertain as to which of these approaches for temporal lobe epilepsy is better in terms of seizure control.[5] Hence, surgeons chose between the two surgical strategies of standard temporal lobectomy and SAH based on their comfort with the procedure.

Major complications that can occur during temporal lobe surgery include injury to the internal carotid artery, anterior choroidal artery, lenticulostriate arteries, third nerve, the large draining vein of the temporal lobe (vein of Labbe), or the brain stem. Damage to these structures can cause devastating neurological deficits. This again stresses the need for the neurosurgeon performing the procedure to have focused training in these procedures in a center having a dedicated epilepsy surgery program. Some of the neurological deficits that are seen following temporal lobe resection which are relatively less morbid include sensory aphasia due to injury to the Wernicke's area and contralateral homonymous superior quadrantinopia due to injury to the Meyer's loop component of the optic radiation.

A study done at Sree Chitra Tirunal Institute for Medical Sciences and Technology, Trivandrum showed that the 50.2% patient had complete resolution of seizures including aura and 77.9% had Engel Class I seizures with no disabling seizures which was comparable to seizure outcome from other centers.

LESIONAL EPILEPSY SURGERY

Anatomically, these lesions can be identified anywhere in the brain (Fig. 2). The seizure semiology depends on the location of the lesion. Surgical removal of these lesions is essential for reduction of seizures. Lesions located in a noneloquent, accessible region of the brain are relatively less risky to resect in the hands of an experienced epilepsy surgeon. When they are located within or near eloquent regions, removal of these lesions becomes challenging. In such situations, intraoperative neurophysiological studies as mentioned earlier in this chapter are done to identify the eloquent brain and the epileptic foci. Some patients are selected for "awake surgery" which helps to assess intraoperatively the integrity of the motor tracts and speech centers during resection of the lesions (Fig. 3). Use of neuronavigation, neurorobot, laser thermocoagulation, and performing the procedure in intraoperative MRI suites helps to improve precision during these procedures. All these are done with an idea to maximize resection of the epileptic lesion and minimize postoperative neurological deficits. Generally, the seizure outcome

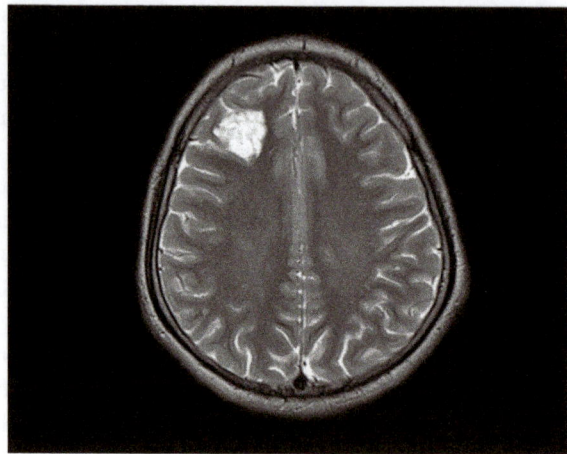

FIG. 2: Axial magnetic resonance imaging of the brain showing a right frontal dysembryoplastic neuroepithelial tumor in a patient with intractable seizures

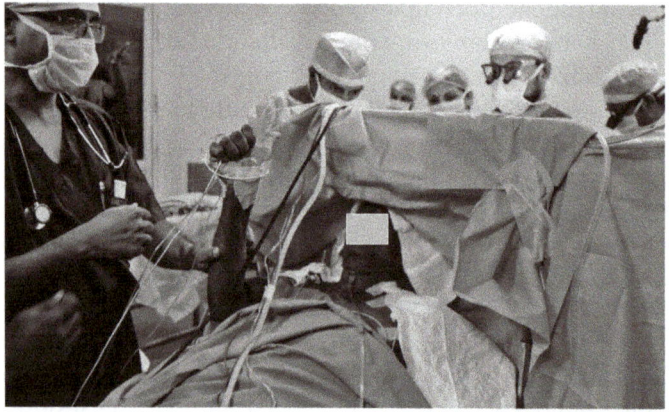

FIG. 3: Theater set up for awake craniotomy showing testing motor power of upper limb by the anesthesia team while the neurosurgical team resects the eloquent brain

for lesional epilepsy is less favorable compared to surgery for MTS or hemispherotomy.

HEMISPHERECTOMY AND HEMISPHEROTOMY

These procedures are done for patients with unihemispheric epilepsy. The underlying lesions in hemispheric epilepsy are multilobar cortical dysplasias, Rasmussen's encephalitis, Sturge Weber syndrome, and ischemic vascular insults.[6]

The first surgical technique described for unihemispheric epilepsy was the anatomic hemispherectomy.[7] The procedure involved removal of one entire hemisphere (Figs 4 and 5). Hemispherectomy later went out of favor due to development of fatal complications like superficial cerebral hemosiderosis (SCH) secondary to creation of a large cavity after removal of the hemisphere.[8] Patients with SCH develop an intracranial space occupying lesion secondary to multiple micro bleeds into the cavity. This later forms a mass that gradually increases in size and kills the patient secondary to raised intracranial pressure. Later, various modifications of techniques evolved with the idea of maximizing disconnection and minimizing removal of brain. One of the notable techniques was the functional hemispherectomy described by Rasmussen.[9] This involved removal of the motor cortex and the temporal lobe and disconnecting the two cerebral hemispheres by a callosotomy. Later, the concept of hemispherotomy became popular that involved disconnecting white mater tracts retaining the cerebral hemisphere as such without disrupting its blood supply. The primary idea of this procedure was to prevent development of a large cavity as seen following hemispherectomy, thus preventing the development of SCH. There are various modifications of this technique.[10,6] Minimally invasive (key hole) endoscopic techniques[11] and endoscope assisted hemispherotomy[12] techniques are now becoming popular. The seizure freedom reported following hemispherotomy techniques is about 77% with low incidence of mortality and morbidity.[6] All these hemispherotomy techniques have comparable excellent seizure outcome with relatively low incidence and less severe complications compared to anatomic hemispherectomy.[7]

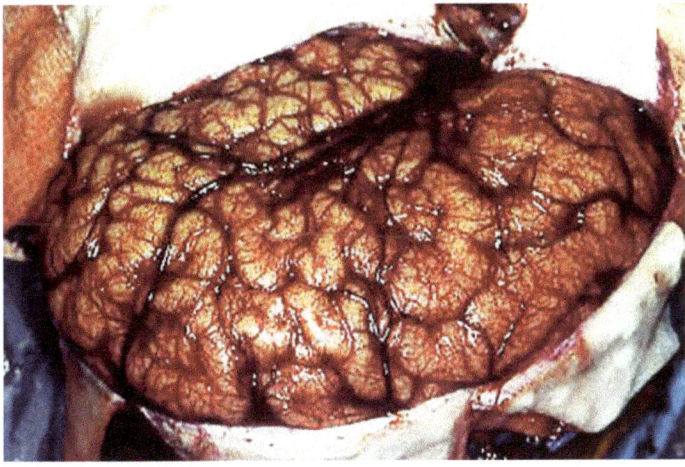

FIG. 4: Intraoperative picture showing exposure of the left hemisphere before hemispherectomy

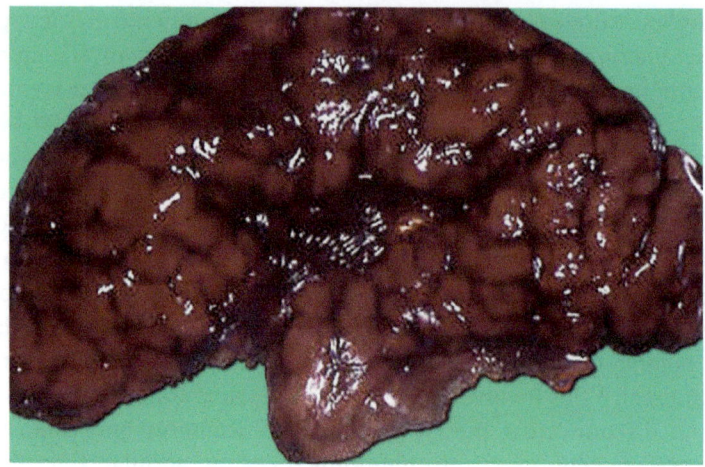

FIG. 5: Intraoperative picture showing the removed left hemisphere after hemispherectomy

HYPOTHALAMIC HAMARTOMAS

Hypothalamic hamartomas (HH) are rare developmental malformations that can cause disabling intractable seizures.[13] Gelastic seizures are the signature of HH, however, other refractory seizure types are also common in these lesions.[14] Gelastic seizures are characterized by repeated short lasting seizures, with initial emotionless laughter or grimacing or rarely vocalization similar to a cry. Other seizure types that can be seen in HH include generalized tonic clonic seizures, drop attacks, complex partial seizures, or atypical absences.[14] Age of onset of these lesions is in the childhood or the neonatal period. The clinical course of HH is often progressive and associated with severe endocrine disturbances, precocious puberty, and cognitive, behavioral, and psychiatric manifestations.[14] These lesions are microscopically made of disordered collection of neurons, glial cells, and fiber bundles. Hypothalamic hamartomas do not have a tendency for neoplastic transformation. They arise from the region of mammillary body or tuber cinerium and the floor of the third ventricle.[14] In the most severe form of seizures in HH, patients go into a state of progressive encephalitic encephalopathy. In the past, it was thought that the seizure onset in HH was from the neocortical region, however, recent studies show that these lesions have intrinsic epileptogenesis.[14]

These lesions can be seen on CT scans or MRI scans. When small, these lesions can be seen attached to the floor of the third ventricle. Large lesions extend beyond this region to the suprasellar cisterns (Fig. 6), interpeduncular region, or the cavity of the third ventricle.

Seizure outcome has been found to be favorable with surgical resection of these lesions.[14] Surgical approaches include microsurgical or endoscopic

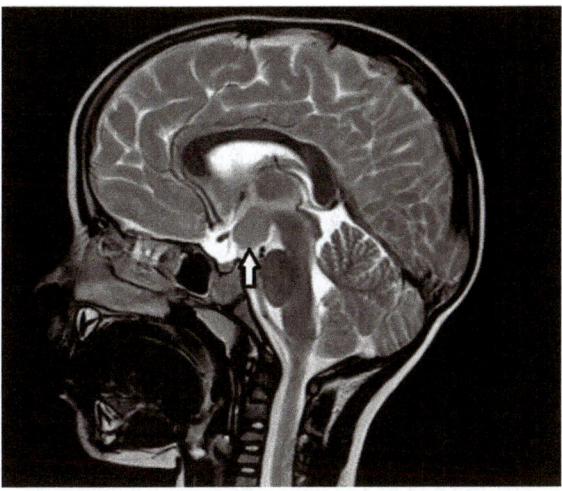

FIG. 6: Sagittal image showing a hypothalamic hamartoma arising in the floor of third ventricle and extending to the suprasellar cistern

resection, radiosurgery, and radiofrequency ablation.[15] Delalande et al.[16] have classified HH into four groups based on its anatomic location. Based on this classification, surgeons can plan the choice of surgical approach. Surgically, these lesions can either be totally removed or disconnected.[16] In a series of 17 patients surgically treated by Delelande, relief of all types of seizures was seen in 8 patients and 7 patients had about 80–90% reduction in seizures.[16] Radiosurgery has also shown almost similar promising results.[15,16]

CORPUS CALLOSOTOMY

Corpus callosotomy (CC) involves sectioning of the corpus callosum including the anterior commissure. The principle of this procedure is to interrupt interhemispheric propagation of seizures. This is under the assumption that corpus callosum is primarily responsible for bilateral synchrony of spike and wave discharges. The procedure is found to be very useful when medically intractable atonic seizures or "drop attacks" are the predominant clinical presentation. Corpus callosotomy can either be total (disconnection of the whole corpus callosum) or partial (partial disconnection of the corpus callosum).[17] Partial callosotomy can be either in the anterior or posterior aspect.[18] Total callosotomy is associated with disconnection syndrome which may improve partially after the procedure. The extent of callosal resection is proportional to the deterioration of cognitive status and a favorable seizure reduction following the procedure. Larger clinical series have shown a favorable seizure outcome following total callosotomy as compared to partial callosotomies.[19] Still, some centers prefer partial callosotomy as a first option considering the lower incidence of cognitive sequelae. If seizures do not improve after partial callosotomy, they proceed with a total callosotomy. Classically, the procedure is done with a microscope; however, endoscopic callosotomy has been described.[18,20] The outcome following CC is favorable even though it is not as high as for mesial temporal lobe surgery or hemispherotomy. A recently published article from Mayo Clinic analyzing 50 patients showed complete resolution of seizures in 40% patients.[21] In the recent past, with the introduction of less invasive and less morbid vagal nerve stimulators, the number of CC that are being performed has decreased dramatically.[22]

VAGAL NERVE STIMULATORS

The vagal nerve stimulator (VNS) was approved in Europe in 1994 and in the United States in 1997 for treating drug-resistant epilepsy in adults and adolescents above the age of 12 years. The device consists of a programmed implantable pulse generator placed in the infraclavicular region in a subcutaneous plane that is connected to the left vagal nerve with electrodes. The optimal stimulation parameters are adjusted after implantation. It has a hand held wand which can activate or deactivate the device. The exact mechanism of action of VNS is unknown and is believed to act by activating various centers of the brain stem, hypothalamus, and forebrain. Complications of VNS are mild generally and include hoarseness of voice, cough, voice change, and breathlessness. The major advantage of the procedure is that it is less invasive and its disadvantage is the high cost. Clinical studies have shown improvement in the quality of life[23,24] and reduction in seizure frequency[25] after VNS.

MULTIPLE SUBPIAL TRANSECTIONS

Multiple subpial transections (MST) is indicated in patients with pharmaco-resistant focal seizures involving eloquent regions of the brain.[26] The underlying principle of MST is that seizures propagate through both horizontal and vertical neuronal networks of the brain. The procedure involves making multiple vertical cuts on the involved region of the brain, thus interrupting the horizontal networks. The procedure thus helps reduce seizures with less chance for neurological deficits. The procedure has shown to achieve seizure freedom in 46% of patients with associated transient motor deficits indicating its acceptable morbidity.[27]

GAMMA KNIFE RADIOSURGERY

The procedure involves delivery of very high dose of radiation to the target with relatively less dose to the surrounding brain thus reducing the incidence of post operative cognitive deficits. The advantage of this type of focused radiation is its usage in patients in whom resective procedures are contraindicated due to associated comorbidities. The major disadvantage however is its delay in onset of action which takes 12–24 months after the treatment.[28] Prospective randomized control, the ROSE (Radiosurgery or open surgery for epilepsy) trial is under way to study the effectiveness of radiosurgery over open resective surgeries for pharmacoresistant epilepsies.[28]

DEEP BRAIN STIMULATION

Numerous regions of the brain have been studied to analyze the usefulness of their stimulation for control of drug-resistant seizures. The regions studied are the caudate nucleus, hippocampus, subthalamic nucleus, and the thalamus.[28] A randomized double blind study, Stimulation of Anterior Nucleus of the Thalamus for Epilepsy (SANTE), in 2010 studied the effectiveness of deep brain stimulation in patients with intractable seizures.[29] The study showed that 54% of patients achieved more than or equal to 50% reduction in seizures, the result of which was comparable to that of VNS. Deep brain stimulation of the anterior nucleus of thalamus is currently considered an adjunctive treatment for refractory epilepsy in Europe and Canada, however, this is not approved by the United States Food and Drug Administration.

CONCLUSION

Surgical treatment of epilepsy is complex that involves team work from multiple subspecialties. Patients with pharmacoresistant epilepsies should be referred to a comprehensive epilepsy program. The key to success of epilepsy surgery is proper selection of patients and demonstration of clinico-radiologic and electrophysiologic concordance. If properly selected for surgery, they yield excellent seizure outcome. Some of the surgical procedures have excellent seizure outcome close to 80%. Use of newer gadgets in neurosurgery and with finer microsurgical techniques, these procedures can be performed with excellent seizure control and reduced rate of complications.

REFERENCES

1. Engel J, Jr. Surgery for seizures. N Engl J Med. 1996;334:647-52.
2. Barkovich AJ, Rowley HA, Andermann F. MR in partial epilepsy: value of high-resolution volumetric techniques. AJNR Am J Neuroradiol. 1995;16:339-43.
3. Falconer MA, Taylor DC. Surgical treatment of drug-resistant epilepsy due to mesial temporal sclerosis. Etiology and significance. Arch Neurol. 1968;19:353-61.
4. Bahuleyan B, Fisher W, Robinson S, Cohen AR. Endoscopic transventricular selective amygdalohippocampectomy: cadaveric demonstration of a new operative approach. World Neurosurg. 2013;80:178-82.

5. Clusmann H, Schramm J, Kral T, Helmstaedter C, Ostertun B, Fimmers R, et al. Prognostic factors and outcome after different types of resection for temporal lobe epilepsy. J Neurosurg. 2002;97:1131-41.
6. Delalande O, Bulteau C, Dellatolas G, Fohlen M, Jalin C, Buret V, et al. Vertical parasagittal hemispherotomy: surgical procedures and clinical long-term outcomes in a population of 83 children. Neurosurgery. 2007;60:ONS19-32; discussion ONS32.
7. Bahuleyan B, Robinson S, Nair AR, Sivanandapanicker JL, Cohen AR. Anatomic hemispherectomy: historical perspective. World Neurosurg. 2013;80:396-8.
8. Oppenheimer DR, Griffith HB. Persistent intracranial bleeding as a complication of hemispherectomy. J Neurol Neurosurg Psychiatry. 1966;29:229-40.
9. Rasmussen T. Hemispherectomy for seizures revisited. Can J Neurol Sci. 1983;10:71-8.
10. Villemure JG, Mascott CR. Peri-insular hemispherotomy: surgical principles and anatomy. Neurosurgery. 1995;37:975-81.
11. Bahuleyan B, Manjila S, Robinson S, Cohen AR. Minimally invasive endoscopic transventricular hemispherotomy for medically intractable epilepsy: a new approach and cadaveric demonstration. J Neurosurg Pediatr. 2010;6:536-40.
12. Chandra SP, Tripathi M. Endoscopic epilepsy surgery: Emergence of a new procedure. Neurol India. 2015;63:571-82.
13. Rao MB, Radhakrishnan K. Is epilepsy surgery possible in countries with limited resources? Epilepsia. 41 Suppl 4:S31-4.
14. Mittal S, Mittal M, Montes JL, Farmer JP, Andermann F. Hypothalamic hamartomas. Part 1. Clinical, neuroimaging, and neurophysiological characteristics. Neurosurg Focus. 2013;34:E6.
15. Unger F, Schrottner O, Haselsberger K, Korner E, Ploier R, Pendl G. Gamma knife radiosurgery for hypothalamic hamartomas in patients with medically intractable epilepsy and precocious puberty. Report of two cases. J Neurosurg. 2000;92:726-31.
16. Delalande O, Fohlen M. Disconnecting surgical treatment of hypothalamic hamartoma in children and adults with refractory epilepsy and proposal of a new classification. Neurol Med Chir (Tokyo). 2003;43:61-8.
17. Jalilian L, Limbrick DD, Steger-May K, Johnston J, Powers AK, Smyth MD. Complete versus anterior two-thirds corpus callosotomy in children: analysis of outcome. J Neurosurg Pediatr. 2010;6:257-66.
18. Bahuleyan B, Vogel TW, Robinson S, Cohen AR. Endoscopic total corpus callosotomy: cadaveric demonstration of a new approach. Pediatr Neurosurg. 2011;47:455-60.
19. Sakas DE, Phillips J. Anterior callosotomy in the management of intractable epileptic seizures: significance of the extent of resection. Acta Neurochir (Wien). 1996;138:700-7.
20. Tubbs RS, Smyth MD, Salter G, Doughty K, Blount JP: Eyebrow incision with supraorbital trephination for endoscopic corpus callosotomy: a feasibility study. Childs Nerv Syst 20:188-191, 2004.
21. Bower RS, Wirrell E, Nwojo M, Wetjen NM, Marsh WR, Meyer FB. Seizure outcomes after corpus callosotomy for drop attacks. Neurosurgery. 2013;73:993-1000.
22. Polkey CE. Alternative surgical procedures to help drug-resistant epilepsy - a review. Epileptic Disord. 2003;5:63-75.
23. Cramer JA. Exploration of Changes in Health-Related Quality of Life after 3 Months of Vagus Nerve Stimulation. Epilepsy Behav. 2001;2:460-5.
24. Handforth A, DeGiorgio CM, Schachter SC, Uthman BM, Naritoku DK, Tecoma ES, et al. Vagus nerve stimulation therapy for partial-onset seizures: a randomized active-control trial. Neurology. 1988;51:48-55.
25. Spanaki MV, Allen LS, Mueller WM, Morris GL, 3rd. Vagus nerve stimulation therapy: 5-year or greater outcome at a university-based epilepsy center. Seizure. 2004;13:587-90.
26. Morrell F, Whisler WW, Bleck TP. Multiple subpial transection: a new approach to the surgical treatment of focal epilepsy. J Neurosurg. 1989;70:231-9.

27. Blount JP, Langburt W, Otsubo H, Chitoku S, Ochi A, Weiss S, et al. Multiple subpial transections in the treatment of pediatric epilepsy. J Neurosurg. 2004;100:118-24.
28. Chang EF, Englot DJ, Vadera S. Minimally invasive surgical approaches for temporal lobe epilepsy. Epilepsy Behav. 2015;47:24-33.
29. Fisher R, Salanova V, Witt T, Worth R, Henry T, Gross R, et al. Electrical stimulation of the anterior nucleus of thalamus for treatment of refractory epilepsy. Epilepsia. 2010;51:899-908.

EU GSPR Authorised Reprsentative
Logos Europe, 9 rue Nicolas Poussin
1700, La Rochelle, France
Phone: +33 (0) 6 67 93 73 78
E-mail: contact@logoseurope.eu